MW01200300

Eat Carbs, Look Better Naked

Shed Unwanted Bodyfat and Achieve Greater Health

Jayson Hunter RD, CSCS

Copyright © 2016 Jayson Hunter RD, CSCS

All rights reserved.

ISBN: 1530099676

ISBN-13: 978-1530099672

DEDICATION

I dedicate this book to my family who always sacrifices for me so that I can do what I do and provide help to others that are in need of my knowledge and guidance.

CONTENTS

Introduction

If you've ever perused your local bookstore's shelves for health guidance, you've no doubt noticed an excess of diet books. Each one has a different plan for your guaranteed success, yet they all claim to be *the one that really works*.

Why is that?

The majority of mainstream diets are designed to be followed very strictly –so they work for a while. However, they don't teach you how to maintain your new bodyweight once you reach your goal. As a result, you end up putting the fat back on.

Then the next diet book comes out, you purchase that and start all over again. You might have some success with the next diet, but, again, it doesn't teach you how to eat healthfully for the long term. So, once again, you put the fat back on.

If you're like most dieters, you've repeated this pattern often, each time getting slightly bigger than the time before. Meanwhile, you're ticked off because you can't figure out why you keep gaining the weight back. Now you have a psychological struggle in addition to a physical one!

Sound familiar?

If so, take heart. This diet plan is different from anything you've read or experienced before.

First, this book gets you into the habit of choosing the right foods and eating the right amounts of them. Then it teaches you why you eat the way you do. You'll also discover how to maintain a healthier lifestyle so you don't regain the fat and revert back to the endless pattern of yo-yo dieting you've struggled with for so long.

Feel relieved? I hope so!

The majority of dieters face common stumbling blocks that keep them from their goals. This program is designed to tear down those barriers.

First, I'll guide you through a detailed nutrition plan for 30 days. Following this plan for the next 30 days allows you to break old habits while forming exciting, new ones. Then we'll address how to ensure you maintain the lean, ripped body you're about to achieve.

When You Want to Look Great for a Special Event

Your special event is right around the corner ...

If you're 30 to 60 days away from an important event - such as your wedding, high-school reunion, tropical vacation or big family get-together - start with the 30-day guided nutrition plan as soon as possible. Later, you can follow the other principles in this book to ensure you end your dieting days once and for all and keep looking and feeling great for the rest of your life.

You have time to spare before your special event ...

If your special event is more than 30 to 60 days away, start by following the 30-day guided nutrition plan now, then transition right into the other principles in this book. You'll start off with the right mindset for forming healthy habits, so you look and feel your best when your big event finally arrives.

Looking Forward to a New You

Down the road, if you ever feel the need to re-focus on your diet or re-form good habits, simply go back to the 30-day nutrition plan outlined in this book. However, I don't advise making it your all-purpose eating approach. Truth is, once you get the fit body you want and learn the healthy way to eat, you can actually maintain your lean look by following the more general eating principles outlined in this book.

With all this talk about the 30-day nutrition plan, you're probably fearing the worst ... My guess is you're thinking I'm here to tell you to do something insane like eat nasty boiled chicken and dry, tasteless rice cakes all day long.

Not a chance. In fact, you'll get to eat most of your favorite foods. I'm going to teach you how to quickly and safely drop pounds, so you look amazing on the day of your big event or vacation.

Hopefully you've been reading about how bad starvation diets are for you. You've probably read on a health website or in a men's magazine how devastating it is to your metabolism when you don't get proper food and nutrients. Chances are, you know from experience that restricting nutrients makes you feel lousy. Maybe you've cut back on meals as a quick-and-easy way to get rid of extra pounds. Or, you've convinced yourself you can lose weight if you just don't bother with breakfast.

Well, those counterproductive antics are behind you now. You're going to discover the secret methods to radically changing your body in the fastest, safest way possible. The Flexible Carb-Cycling Diet will melt fat from your midsection and wherever else you need it, leaving you with a tighter, more cut-looking body. And you'll finish this book with the wisdom to maintain that look.

During these next 30 days, you will follow a *carb cycling* program that consists of all the proper nutrients – carbs, proteins and fats. Fitness competitors drop weight and lean out their bodies by cutting carbs. However, cutting carbs all the time actually forces your body into starvation mode. We don't want that! This is not a low-carb diet.

It's a *carb cycling* diet. When you cycle your carbohydrate intake, you succeed at losing fat without sending your body into the dreaded starvation mode. Carb cycling means consuming a moderate to low amount of carbohydrates, which promotes your ability to burn calories.

Unlike crash or fad diets, this eating plan puts you on the path to short-term *and* long-term success. Be prepared to maintain your ideal weight for life! In just 30 days, you'll be on the road to having the fit body you've been wanting for so long. Plus, you'll feel confident knowing when your big event is over, you won't pack on the pounds again.

The reason 99% of all diets fail is because they're designed to work only in the short term. Not this one.

I'm here to show you how to turn your short-term success into long-term success with healthy, safe lifestyle change. After the next 30 days, you'll learn the behavioral changes needed to maintain your new, improved bodyweight for the rest of your life.

Are you ready? *Are you excited?* **You should be.**

The new you begins now!

Chapter 1

30 Days To A New You

I'm expecting you might consider this diet a little unusual at first. I'm not going to rehash all the run-of-the-mill stuff you see over and over in magazines. This isn't the regurgitated diet plan every so-called guru out there puts in his or her "best-selling" book.

This program works amazingly well when you follow simple instructions. That's because this plan is based on very advanced information. Still, my goal is to keep everything as basic as possible. I won't confuse or bore you with information you don't need to know. Everything in this book is here because it's what you need to achieve a quick and safe reduction in bodyweight. Period.

To get started, let's look at the basics for the first 30 days:

1. You will be "cycling" your carbohydrate intake. One day will be "high carbs." One day will be "low carbs." Another day will be "no-carbs."

2. Your protein intake will be moderate to high.

3. Your fat intake will be moderate to low.

4. Most of your fat will come from protein sources and fish oils. Your body needs fat to exist, so please do not make the mistake of eliminating fat from your diet. Eliminating fat will *not* help you lose weight quickly and safely.

5. As part of this plan, I do recommend highly researched and 100% safe supplements because they aid your metabolism and improve fat burning. No, they are NOT controversial fat burners such as Ephedra. I wouldn't dream of recommending that.

6. The Flexible Carb-Cycling Diet is based on eating 4-5 times a day. This includes having protein and vegetables at every meal.

I'll get into more detail about all the above points later in this book.

Calorie Needs

On the Flexible Carb-Cycling Diet, you will be determining your calorie needs. But you will only be using these numbers as a reference. Don't worry: You won't be counting calories at every meal or even every day. I know you don't have the time or patience for that. You will only use this calorie formula if you think you may be consuming too much food.

At meals, you'll consume your protein, vegetables and fruit first and your carbs last. Generally, though, by the time you eat your protein, vegetable and fruit you won't be that hungry for many carbs. This helps you avoid over-consuming carbs.

Here is a simple formula for determining your body's daily caloric needs..)

(Note: RMR stands for "Resting Metabolic Rate," a fancy term for your daily caloric needs.)

$$1 \text{ inch} = 0.0254 \text{ meters}$$
$$1 \text{kg} = 2.2 \text{ lbs}$$

Men's Formula for RMR= 293 − (3.8 x age) + (456.4 x height in meters) + (10.12 x weight in kg)

(If you know your lean-body-mass number from a body-fat calculation, use that number as the weight in kg.)

Now multiply your RMR x 0.85 to determine your overall

calories. This is the estimated calories you need to consume every day.

EXAMPLE
36-year-old male, 5' 9" in height, 205 lbs in weight

First, convert height and weight into meters and kilograms in order to use the formula above.

HEIGHT: 5'9" = 69". Convert to meters by multiplying 69 x 0.0254 = **1.752 meters**

WEIGHT: 205 lbs divided by 2.2 = **93 kg**

Now that we've converted height and weight into meters and kilograms, we're ready to determine this person's caloric needs.

RMR= 293 – (3.8 x 36) + (456.4 x 1.752) + (10.12 x 93)

RMR= 293 - 136.8 + 799.6 + 941

RMR= 1,896 calories

1896 x 0.85= 1,612 calories per day

$$191 - (3.8 \times 62) + (456.4 \times 1.727) + (0.12 \times 86.81)$$
$$235.6 + 788.20 + 878.51$$
$$11$$
$$1622.11$$

Women's Formula for RMR

247 – (2.67 x age) + (401.5 x height in meters) + (8.6 x weight in kg)

(If you know your lean-body-mass number from a body-fat calculation, use that number as the weight in kg.)

Now multiply your RMR x 0.85 to determine your overall calories. This is the estimated calories you need to consume every day.

EXAMPLE
34-year-old female, 5' 4" in height, 130 lbs in weight

First, we convert height and weight into meters and kilograms in order to use the formula above.

HEIGHT: 5'4" = 64". Convert to meters by multiplying 64 x 0.0254 = **1.625 meters** 1.727

WEIGHT: 130 lbs divided by 2.2 = **59 kg** 86.81

Now that we've converted height and weight into meters and kilograms, we're ready to determine this person's caloric needs.

RMR= 247- (2.67 x 34) + (401 .5 x 1 .62 5) + (8.6 x 59) RMR= 247- 90.78 + 652.43 + 507.4

RMR= 1316.05

1316.05 x 0.85= 1,118 calories per day   1378 cal.

Determine your own caloric needs using the formula above. Then read on to learn how you will obtain the calories you need, and from what types of foods.

Protein

As I wrote earlier, protein will be a diet staple for the next 30 days, so don't skimp on this nutrient or take it for granted. Your protein choices will be mostly lean, such as eggs whites and salmon, along with a few "medium-fat" proteins like steak and mozzarella cheese.

You'll be eating 4-5 meals, spread out so you eat about every 3 hours during the waking day. Three or 4 of these 5 daily meals will include lean proteins. One or 2 of these meals will contain protein with a slightly higher fat content (see below for examples).

You should eat 1 gram of protein per pound of bodyweight, and no less (see chart below). So for a 205-pound man, the minimum protein intake would be 205 grams of protein each day. Remember, though, this isn't about eating for the sake of eating. You need to eat until you feel full and satisfied, not stuffed.

TIP

Put your fork down while chewing, and don't pick it up until you swallow what's in your mouth.

(Think this little tip is silly? Well, it's one crucial key to controlling your caloric intake. Try it and see.)

Protein sources approved for the Flexible Carb-Cycling Diet:

Lean Protein Sources:

- Chicken or turkey (white meat)
- Tuna fish (canned, in water)
- Lean beef
- Egg whites
- Non-fat cottage cheese
- Fish (shark, salmon, flounder, etc.)
- Shellfish

"Medium-Fat" Protein Sources:

- Chicken or turkey (dark meat)
- Whole eggs
- Cottage cheese (2% or whole)
- Steaks (moderate fat cuts, 20 to 25% fat)
- Other meats (moderate fat, 20 to 25% fat)
- Mozzarella cheese (non-fat or skim)

TIP

When choosing fish for lean protein, ask where the fish comes from. Fish farms are generally safe from contaminants. Many people don't realize store-bought fish is less contaminated than fish caught in the wild.

What equals 1 gram of protein?

1 ounce of meat equals 7 grams of protein.
A 3-ounce piece of meat is the size of a deck of cards. So, it's roughly 21 grams of protein.
1 whole egg (includes yolk) equals 7 grams of protein.
2 egg whites equal roughly 7 grams of protein.

Fats

Let me emphasize again that fat is a necessary nutrient. Your body needs it. Fat provides additional energy reserves, protects vital organs and transports fat-soluble vitamins. It's also a great hunger depressor. It can take up to 3.5 hours to empty fat from the stomach, so dietary fat helps prevent hunger pangs before your next meal. Bottom Line: Don't drop body fat altogether.

You might notice I don't have a list of approved fats for this section. That's because there isn't one per se. You'll get most of the fats you need primarily from the protein choices I've already discussed.

Having said that, I highly suggest you supplement your diet with potent Essential Fatty Acids. Doing so will supply your body with essential fats that keep your metabolism going strong. I'll go into more detail about these supplements later in this book.

Nutrient-Rich Vegetables

Get ready to eat a variety of nutrient-rich vegetables every day. I'm talking about vegetables that are high in fiber and under 50 calories per cup. You should eat at least 1 to 1.5 cups (cooked or raw) of nutrient-rich vegetables at 4 of your 6 daily meals.

Remember, you will eat your vegetables with your protein source *before* you eat any carbohydrates. Like protein, nutrient-rich, high-fiber vegetables help you feel full. By eating your protein and vegetables first - and setting your fork down between bites - you will feel full faster, which prevents you from overeating.

Nutrient-rich vegetables approved for the Flexible Carb-Cycling Diet:

- Broccoli
- Salad (lettuce, romaine, etc.); use non-fat dressing.
- Cabbage
- Green beans
- Spinach
- Zucchini
- Squash
- Red or green pepper
- Asparagus
- Carrots
- Tomatoes
- Cauliflower
- Mushrooms
- Artichoke hearts

Carbohydrates

"Carb cycling" is the critical component of the Flexible Carb-Cycling Diet. This is where you alternate between high-carbohydrate, low-carbohydrate and no-carbohydrate days. And, as I've mentioned, you will consume carbs only after eating your protein, vegetable and fruit requirements for a given meal. It's simple:

Day 1: High Carbs
Day 2: Low Carbs
Day 3: No Carbs
Day 4: High Carbs
Day 5: Low Carbs
Day 6: No Carbs

Day 7: High Carbs (and so on, following that cycle, for 30 days total).

Carbohydrates approved for Flexible Carb-Cycling Diet:

- Sweet potatoes or yams
- Brown rice
- Corn
- Peas
- Legumes (chickpeas, lima beans, lentils, dry beans)
- High-fiber cereals (All Bran, Fiber One, Grape Nuts, Cracklin' Oat Bran, Shredded Wheat)

- Oats and oatmeal (not instant oatmeal)
- Black beans
- 100% wholegrain pasta (Eden, Hodgson Mill, Purity Foods)
- 100% wholegrain bread (Pepperidge Farm, Nature's Path, Nature's Own, Earth Grains)

Let's look at how each of the carb cycles described above will work.

High-Carbohydrate Day

On this day, you will eat all the carbs you like until you reach fullness. Again, you aren't stuffing yourself. You'll already have eaten your protein source, vegetables and fruit, so you shouldn't be too hungry.

Don't feel guilty for eating carbs. They help you melt fat and lose inches. Plus, your body needs the calories from this energy source to prevent your metabolism from slowing down and ruining your weight loss efforts.

As part of these high-carb meals, you will need to eat 1 piece of high-fiber fruit before the carbs. So a meal on this day would look like this:

HIGH-CARB DAY

1 lean or medium-fat protein source
  (depending on which meal of the day)

1 nutrient-rich vegetable

1 high-fiber fruit

High-fiber fruits approved for Flexible Carb-Cycling Diet:

- Raspberries
- Strawberries
- Blackberries
- Apple
- Pear
- Prunes
- Orange

Low-Carbohydrate Day

On this day, you will eat the same types of carbs as on the high-carbohydrate day but you will more closely limit your carb intake to only 2 of the 4-5 meals (which you don't have to do on the high-carb days). Again, consume your protein and vegetable servings first. Then eat 1 gram per pound of your bodyweight of an "approved" carbohydrate source for the day. Divide this carbohydrate total by 2 and eat ½ of your total carbs at

2 of your 4-5 meals for the day. This includes your piece of approved high-fiber fruit at each meal (to be eaten before the carbs).

I'll give you an example of how this works. A 205-pound man would consume 205 grams of "approved" carbs on "low-carb" days, so that's 51.25 grams of carbs spread out over 4 meals. Remember, you eat carbs at only 4 of the 6 daily meals. The remaining 2 meals of the day would be "no carbs," just protein and nutrient-rich vegetables.

TIP

Exercise helps you lose weight and increase health. If you work out (and I strongly suggest you do), consume one of your 4 "carb" meals after a workout.

No-Carb Day

When I say "no-carb," I mean no added carbohydrates at all. You will still get a few carbs by eating the nutrient-rich vegetables. But you definitely will not be eating fruit or any of the Flexible Carb-Cycling Diet -approved carbohydrates.

Each meal on these days consists of your recommended protein intake along with 1 to 1.5 cups of vegetables (see approved list in Vegetables section). Also, make sure you take your high quality Essential Fatty Acid supplement to obtain the fats your body needs for good health and optimal metabolism.

I realize that it might be difficult in the beginning to forgo all forms of starchy carbohydrate. Your body is probably used to them, and you'll feel hungry without them. But this no-carb day is crucial to your success. And keep in mind that the very next day is a high-carb day! Something to look forward to.

Now, there's one loophole on this day. If you exercise on a no-carb day, you get an exemption. Research shows that consuming a quick-digesting carbohydrate and protein drink within 60 minutes of working out is very beneficial. So I recommend you do just that. Ideally, make it a post-workout recovery shake that consists of around 30 grams of carbohydrates and 15 grams of protein. So, to recap, you get to have one post-workout carb source on a no-carb day, but only if you workout, of course.

Here is a quick sample of a no-carb day:

NO-CARB DAY

Meal 1: 3 egg whites, 1 yolk omelet, 1 oz. mozzarella cheese, 1/2 cup spinach

Meal 2: 1 oz. almonds, 1 cup baby carrots

Meal 3: 4 oz. chicken breast with seasoning of your choice, salad with approved vegetables and non-fat dressing, 1 hard boiled egg.

(Workout session followed by your fourth meal.)

Meal 4: Post-workout drink

Meal 5: 5 oz. lean beef, 1 cup broccoli, 1/2 cup

Guidelines for No-Carb Days

It's important that you don't stray from the prescribed program. It was created this way for very scientific reasons. Please DO NOT assume if you incorporate more "no-carb" days you will get faster or better results. You won't. I don't know how to be more blunt than that. The reason you are "cycling" these high, low and zero carbohydrate days is so your body doesn't trigger its starvation response. Instead, it keeps running at full efficiency (meaning it burns more calories). More is not always better, and this is one of those instances. Trust me, if you follow the Flexible Carb-Cycling Diet to the letter, you will see amazing results.

So don't get too hung up on tracking calories. Earlier, we estimated your calories only so you could use that value as a guideline to make sure you are not eating too little or too much. If you put your fork down between bites and carefully monitor when you feel satisfied and not stuffed, you should never have to measure your caloric intake. Your low-carb day will be about equal to your caloric estimation. Your high-carb day will be a little higher, and your no-carb day a little lower. There is no need to measure your calories on your high-carb or no-carb days.

Base your serving sizes on how full you feel, and not on what the calories or grams say. Simply follow the guidelines listed above, in the order they are suggested. If you are the type who needs to have a reference point to work from, record how many grams of carbs and protein you eat for the first few days until you feel comfortable with how much food equals your protein and carbohydrate total for each day.

Since we're on the topic of monitoring your eating, let's talk about tracking your progress. Weigh yourself only once every 7 to 10 days. I suggest you weigh yourself in the morning after a no-carb day. And consider taking other measurements, as well. Measure your hips, waist, legs, arms and chest before and after the Flexible Carb-Cycling Diet.

TIP

The process of cycling carbohydrates may cause your bodyweight to fluctuate frequently in the beginning. This is due to water loss and gain.

Days Leading up to Your Event

In the last few days leading up to your event, you will change your carb cycle to a high, low, low, no-carb cycle. So if your event is on a Saturday your schedule would look like this:

Tuesday = High carb

Wednesday = Low carb

Thursday = Low carb

Friday = No carb

Saturday = Day of the event (make it a low-carb day, if possible)

This will optimize the Flexible Carb-Cycling Diet and have you looking lean and muscular on the big day.

3 Important Pieces of Advice

1) As I suggested above, on the day of the event, I recommend you select low carbs to help you look your best all day long.

2) Drink plenty of water. For the duration of the Flexible Carb-Cycling Diet, drink 1 oz. of water for every 1.5 to 2 pounds of bodyweight per day. Staying hydrated helps ensure the best results possible.

3) I want to stress that the Flexible Carb-Cycling Diet is just the beginning of your body's transformation. This is NOT a diet to follow for the rest of your life. But it is a huge stepping stone to a stronger-looking, happier and healthier you. After the 30 days of carb cycling, there is simply no reason for you to gain back the unhealthy fat you've worked so hard to lose.

Once you've completed the 30-day nutrition plan explained in this chapter, use the information provided in the rest of this book to make the most of your hard work and success.

Chapter 2:

Here's To Your Health: How to Stay Strong For Life

After you complete the first 30 days, it's time to apply your successes to a lifetime of healthful eating. Just think - you'll never have to diet again.

While you're learning the principles needed to maintain your great physique, I suggest you continue to follow an eating plan similar to your low-carb days. With one exception: Eat an approved carbohydrate for *every* meal of the day (i.e., all 4-5 meals) instead of only 2 meals in the day. For example, if you weighed 205 pounds, you would eat 205 grams of carbs over 4 daily meals (that's about 51 grams of carbs at each meal).

Once you learn the principles in the rest of this book, you'll naturally follow a similar meal plan to the low-carb days without having to calculate everything. You'll have the knowledge to eat the right types and amounts of food. Read on to find out how simple behavioral changes will help you look your best for the rest of your life.

Boosting Your Metabolism

One of the main keys to losing body fat and keeping it off is boosting your metabolism. You can do this a few ways.

Eat Often:

One way is to eat frequently throughout the day. By frequently, I mean eating 4-5 times a day. Every time you eat, your metabolism elevates due to the energy it takes to digest food. Eating frequent meals boosts metabolism all day long, so you burn more calories.

Conversely, if you eat infrequently or go too long between meals, your brain tells your body to slow down, which burns fewer overall calories. This is your body's way of protecting itself by conserving calories for future use and survival.

Some people call this process "starvation mode." In starvation mode, your body burns carbs and protein in your muscles for energy, and it stores the fat. The result? Less muscle mass compared to fat mass, which means a lower resting metabolic rate and fewer calories burned.

Plus, if you limit calories by eating less food or less frequently, you'll feel hungry and deprived. This causes you to eat when you shouldn't - and eat the wrong foods.

Eat Well:

Another way to boost your metabolism is by eating the right types of foods, such as protein. Protein is a metabolically costly food, meaning it requires more calories to digest and utilize protein compared to carbohydrate. I'll talk in more detail about this when we get to the chapter called "Yes, It's True: You Are What You Eat."

Build Muscle:

Another way to boost metabolism is with strength training. Of course, that's another book in itself! Just know that targeted strength training and cardio workouts can increase the number of calories you burn by an additional 300 to 600 calories per day.

In summary, here are some ways to boost your metabolism:

- Eat 4-5 times a day
- Increase your protein intake
- Exercise a minimum of 5 hours a week, including 2 hours of strength training per week

The Emotional Side of Eating: How to Develop the Right Mindset

Food stirs up emotions. We eat when we're stressed and nervous. We do it even when we know we have eaten too much. Why does food control so much of our lives?

Because we let it!

We allow ourselves to think food makes everything better and weight loss will solve all our problems. This leads to self-defeating thoughts and feelings that hold us back from succeeding.

The solution is to restructure thinking processes so they are more constructive. For example, let's say you eat a candy bar from the vending machine. But you know you *should have* eaten a handful of almonds instead. So you conclude you've blown it for the rest of the day. You think, "Why continue eating well today since I already screwed up with that candy bar?"

When you restructure your thoughts to be more constructive, you avoid feeling defeated. You know the candy bar wasn't the best choice, but you recommit to eating more healthfully at lunch and dinner. That way, you still end the day on a healthy note.

Make it a priority to think more constructively. If you feel like you've failed every time something isn't perfect, you will never succeed. Weight loss is hard enough as it is! Being prepared to handle the inevitable bumps in the road is what determines your success.

Realize that you won't lose weight every day, and there will be times when you overindulge. Guess what? That's normal. It's part of the weight-loss cycle. Just keep moving toward your goals.

Still, even with the right mindset, there's no denying that certain foods soothe us. We crave them. We feel calm and relaxed when we eat them. Essentially, we eat because it makes us happy and feel good inside.

Researchers have shown that foods containing sugar and fat increase the production of endorphins, which are the body's "feel good" chemicals. This may be one reason why so many people gravitate toward sweets and desserts rather than vegetables and protein.

To conquer this psychological challenge, you need to create the right mindset, which includes controlling what you eat. Foods that contain sugar and fat are not what's making you fat. What is? You eat too much of sugar and fat!

So what's the solution?

First, stay positive at all times, reinforcing that you're committed to making the right food choices for your body to be healthier.

Second, set an attainable, realistic goal with a timeline (see below for more details). This focuses your mind on working toward that goal. Remind yourself every day what your goal is. This helps you form a mindset toward reaching that goal.

SMART Goals

By now, you have goals in mind for what you want to achieve even if they aren't fully formed yet (that's why you're reading this book). Now it's time to put those goals on paper. Before you do, though, you must learn a bit about proper goal-setting.

A goal needs to meet the SMART criteria to be realistic and attainable. If we didn't set SMART goals, well then, we could just create any goal, such as becoming a millionaire with a pro athlete's body!

Here's how setting a SMART goal works. It must be:

S = Specific

M = Measurable

A = Attainable

R = Realistic

T = Timely

Specific means you describe specifically what the goal is, using a what, why and how method. For example:

>   *WHAT* are you going to do? Describe descriptively what you want to achieve or do.

>   *WHY* is this important to do now? What is your ultimate goal? Be specific.

>   *HOW* are you going to meet this goal, and when?

Your goals should be very specific, clear and easy. Instead of setting a goal to lose weight (which is too general), set a specific goal to lose 4 inches off your waist or fit into a size large shirt instead of the XL.

Measurable is where you track your progress so you see changes occur in a tangible way. What will you see when you reach your goal? Describe the specific target to be measured, such as, "I want to see a 1-inch space between my current jeans and my stomach before my birthday."

People who measure their progress tend to stay on track, reach their target dates and experience better success and fulfillment than those who don't. When you feel good about reaching a goal, you're especially inspired to shoot for another.

Attainable means you need to develop attitudes, abilities, skills and the financial capacity to reach your goal. You figure out what it takes to achieve your goal, and what will make it attainable.

Goals that are too lofty – like the millionaire pro athlete example from above - are virtually unattainable. Even with the best of intentions, you will give up on unattainable goals before too long.

A SMART goal is challenging, requiring a real commitment from you. But it's also *reachable*. For instance, if you aim to lose 30 lbs in 1 week, you're doomed for failure. That's unrealistic. However, setting a goal to lose 2 lbs per week for the next 3 weeks is attainable.

Realistic means a goal is "doable." If you work hard and do the right things, your goal will become a reality.

Having a plan for how you will reach your goal helps make it more realistic. For example, your goal might be to drink 8 ounces of water, 11 times a day. That's doable.

Timely refers to setting deadlines. To have a clear target to work toward, you need a date by which your goal will be achieved. This timeline must be attainable and realistic. Saying you'll get to your goal some time in the future is too vague. It holds you back from reaching your goal.

Once you have created SMART goals, you will be able to clearly see the steps needed to successfully achieve them.

Inches, Pounds & Percentages: How to Track Your Results

The Flexible Carb-Cycling Diet is a results-based program, meaning you need to measure progress and results. Therefore, you'll be re-assessing your body fat and circumference measurements every 3 to 4weeks. The results will determine what changes need to be made to your meal plan, if any.

The following guide is designed to teach you how to take reliable and accurate recordings of your body fat. Record these measurements in the excel document included with the online bonuses for this book to determine your body-fat calculation. https://mealplans101.com/online-bonuses/

You may also use the manual calculation provided in this

chapter and record it on a spreadsheet, or wherever you find it easiest to record information about your body composition.

Circumference Measurements

You will take circumference measurements every 3 to 4weeks to evaluate your progress and determine if you need to make adjustments to your diet and exercise program.

First, purchase a reliable body circumference measuring tape. You can find them at most fitness equipment stores or online at www.quickmedical.com/fitness/handheld/index.html.

Once you have your measuring tape, take measurements of the following key areas for men. Women I have listed your areas for measurement below these.

Abdominal circumference: Place the tape around your midsection so it's level with your navel (bellybutton). Record the measurement onto your excel spreadsheet or other tracking tool.

Chest: Place the tape measure around your chest so it's level with your nipple line. You'll need to measure with your arms at your sides, so ask a partner to help you.

Arms: Measure the largest circumference of the right

arm. Once you have found this point, measure from the top of the shoulder down to the largest part of the right arm. Record the distance, so you can measure at the same spot every time.

Thigh: Measure the largest circumference of the right thigh. Once you have found this point, measure from the top of the kneecap up to the thigh site. Record the distance so you can measure at the same spot every time.

Women's Measurement Locations:

Abdominal circumference: Place the tape around your midsection so it's level with your navel (bellybutton). Record the measurement onto your excel spreadsheet or other tracking tool.

Waist: Measure the narrowest part of your torso between the xiphoid process (bony space in the center of your chest between each side of the ribcage) and your bellybutton.

Hips: Measure the largest circumference of the buttocks above the fold between your butt and leg. Also, take a measurement from underneath your armpit down to this site so you can measure at the same spot every time.

Thigh: Measure the largest circumference of the right thigh. Once you have found this point, measure from the top of the kneecap up to the thigh site. Record the distance so you can measure at the same spot every time.

Record these measurements on a spreadsheet (there's one included with this book called "Body-Fat Calculator"), or other tracking tool. Gauge your progress every 3 to 4 weeks.

Body-Fat Percentage

There are a number of ways you can measure your body-fat percentage, but a lot of them are costly or hard to come by. So we're going to stick with the easiest system for measuring body fat at home – with a skin-fold caliper. You will use this simple, cost-effective device to measure the thickness of the skin at certain locations on your body. Then, based on these measurements, you will estimate your body-fat percentage.

Step 1.

First, purchase a pair of inexpensive skin-fold calipers. You can find them at fitness stores or online from a company called Accu-measure: http://accufitness.com. This company makes a quality pair of skin-fold calipers for a reasonable price.

Step 2.

Find a partner. There is a method for measuring just 1 site on yourself, which we will discuss later. However, the 3-site skin-fold method, which requires the help of a partner, is more accurate. The latter method uses skin folds at 3 sites on the body to determine your body-fat percentage.

Step 3.

Practice. There may be a margin of error due to measuring mistakes, so make sure you and your partner practice first to produce the most accurate measurements possible. With practice, your measurements will become very consistent. See below for guidelines on how to perform each measurement.

Step 4.

Record your results by measuring each site 3 times. Once you have measured each site 3 times, take the average of all 3 numbers, so you're left with one value. Your 3 measurements for each site should be within 10% of each other. If they are not, continue taking measurements of that site until you get 3 numbers that are the closest to each other. I suggest you measure yourself at the same time of day (every 3 to 4 weeks). This reduces error.

Below are guidelines to help you create consistent measurements.

- Take all measurements on the right side of the body every time.

- Pull the skin away from the body to separate it from the muscle. Don't pinch extremely hard. Just squeeze enough to pull the skin away from the body, then place the calipers ½ inch below your thumb and finger.

- Continue holding the skin while taking the measurement.

- Wait a few seconds before re-taking the measurement. Complete each skin-fold site once and then return to measure each site 2 more times. This will allow the skin to recover before taking another measurement.

- Take a minimum of 3 measurements at each site, then determine an average.

Step 5.

Input the skin-fold numbers. Plug the numbers into the excel formula provided with this book.

Measurement Techniques for Each Skin-Fold Site

Now I'll tell you the 3 sites to measure, and how to do it. Note: The measurement sites are different for men and women. I'll focus on the 3 sites for males: umbilical/abdominal site (bellybutton), chest and thigh. Refer to the descriptions and illustrations below to guide you. Women's sites will be listed below these.

Site 1: Abdominal

The landmark to measure is 1 inch directly to the left of, and in line with, the bellybutton. Pinch and measure a vertical fold of skin, as demonstrated in the photograph below. Making an X, as shown, helps with accuracy.

Site 2: Chest

This landmark is on the diagonal line between the armpit and nipple. Find the halfway point between the armpit and nipple, then measure a diagonal fold.

Site 3: Thigh

Select a vertical fold on the front of the thigh, midway between the kneecap and inguinal crease (the inguinal crease is the line where the leg inserts into the trunk at the hip). Measure this distance and mark the midpoint. Pinch the skin fold at that mark to take a measurement.

As discussed, measure each site 3 times. Input the average numbers for each site into the excel spreadsheet (called "Body-Fat Calculator") that comes with this book.

The 3 sites for females: triceps (back of upper arm), suprailium (hip) and thigh. Refer to the descriptions below to guide you.

Site 1: Triceps

This site is located on the back of the upper arm, halfway between the elbow and the bony point on the top of your shoulder. Mark the halfway point with a marker, then pinch a vertical fold of skin as demonstrated.

Site 2: Suprailium

The suprailiac site is the area just above the frontal angle of the iliac crest (or, in plain language, the hip). To measure this landmark, find the front of the hip, then select a diagonal fold of skin approximately 0.5 to 1 inch above that point.

Site 3: Thigh

Select a vertical fold on the front of the thigh, midway between the kneecap and inguinal crease (the inguinal crease is the line where the leg inserts into the trunk at the hip). Measure this distance and mark the midpoint. Pinch the skin fold at that mark to take a measurement.

As discussed, measure each site 3 times. Input the average numbers for each site into the excel spreadsheet (called "Body-Fat Calculator") that comes with this book in the online resources at https://mealplans101.com/online-bonuses/

Keep a Food Journal

Who needs to keep a food log? Anyone who wants to experience success with weight loss, that's who.

Do you write checks without a clue about how much money is in your checking account? Not if you want to avoid bouncing checks. Do you start driving to a destination without any idea how to get there? No. You'd likely drive around in circles.

Well, what about recording what you eat?

If you don't keep track of what you eat, you don't know if you're eating too much or too little of the right foods or the wrong foods. Most importantly, you don't know what to change from one day to the next to improve your meal plan and overall health.

If I ate the same way for 3 months and didn't lose a single pound, I'd want to know what I should change in my diet to start losing weight. If I didn't write it down, I wouldn't have the answer in front of me.

A food journal helps you learn how much you eat, what you eat, when you eat and possibly *why* you've adopted certain eating patterns. It helps you track calories, so it's easier to make changes.

The average person underestimates his or her food consumption by 25%. And research shows that when overweight subjects are asked to recall what they ate in the previous 24 hours, subjects are only able to recall about 50% of the foods and quantities they ate. The reason is, we tend to nibble and graze or aren't conscious of our true portion sizes. Studies by O'Neil and Carels et al. show that self-monitored eating enhances weight loss.

So there you have it - a self-monitoring tool like a food journal makes you aware of what food you eat before it even goes in your mouth. How come? You know you have to write it down if you consume it!

In addition to recording what and how much you eat, use the food journal to record how you feel when you ate that food. Were you very hungry or only slightly hungry? How did you feel after you were finished eating? Use the following scale to help control your portions and become more in tune with your body and satiety.

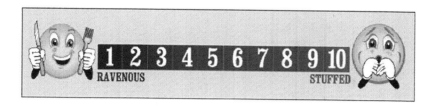

A "1" on the scale means you are so hungry, it's practically making you feel sick. Your stomach aches and grumbles, etc. A "10" on the scale means you're so stuffed you couldn't eat another bite.

As you eat, you should start to feel satisfied and content. This feeling is usually around "5" to "7" on the above scale, and it's the point where you want to stop eating.

Remember my tip from earlier about allowing your body

time to recognize it's had enough food? Set your fork down between bites, chew and swallow before picking up your fork to take another bite.

Once you think you've reached "5" to "7" on the scale above, you might want to stop eating for 10 to 15 minutes. If you're still hungry after 10 to 15 minutes, eat a little more. More than likely, though, you will decide you've had enough. In fact, you may even feel a little fuller than when you first stopped eating because it takes your body time to recognize how much food is in the stomach. This is one reason why it's so easy to overeat.

Social Support

Research shows that enlisting the support of others helps people succeed at weight loss more quickly. People who seek social support may be 42% more likely to lose weight compared to those who do not seek social support. Remember the mindset you are creating ... social support is a significant part of your new mindset. Surround yourself with positive people who will be there to help keep you on track.

Where should your social support come from? Don't assume your family members are the best candidates. Sometimes they are the worst choices! Anyone who has a negative attitude concerning your body weight should not have a role in your social support. Friends or colleagues who also want to lose weight may be good allies because you can work together to keep each other on track.

Exercise

I won't spend a lot of time on this because it's a broad enough topic to fill another book. Bottom line: Exercise is a must, and I don't mean going for a walk. I mean strength training and interval cardio workouts.

Research shows that low-repetition strength training can improve fat loss more than high-rep exercise alone. One study found that subjects who performed 8 repetitions per set of an exercise burned more calories after exercise compared to using 12 repetitions per exercise.

Some people lift weights, but they don't understand how resistance training helps with fat loss. If you want to maximize your metabolism - and get ripped arms, abs and legs while you're at it - you must include high-intensity strength training in your workouts. High-intensity strength training protects your lean muscle mass and increases your fat-burning furnace.

As for cardio exercise, interval training is superior to slow cardio for fat loss because it burns more calories in less time. Researchers at Laval University in Quebec, Canada, conducted a study comparing slow, steady aerobic training with interval training in a fat loss program. The researchers found that the interval-training group lost more fat than the cardio group.

It only takes 3 50-minute workouts a week to start building the body you've always wanted – one that feels and looks fit and lean.

12 "Rules" for Fat Loss Success

At the core of every successful diet plan, fad or nutrition system, there are basic rules for success. Here are the 12 "rules" for fat loss success. You will learn more about each one later in this book.

1. Eat 4 to 5 small meals a day instead of the usual 2 to 3 large meals. Space your meals about 3 hours apart throughout the day. Eating consistently during your waking hours requires your body to spend energy digesting food.

2. Consume whole foods that are high in fiber and low in sugar, such as lean protein (lean beef,

chicken, fish, whey protein), fruits and vegetables (oranges, apples, strawberries, blueberries, broccoli, peppers, asparagus, carrots), nuts (almonds, cashews, walnuts), and whole grains.

3. Eat low-glycemic carbohydrates, such as vegetables, wholegrain products and oatmeal instead of refined, processed carbohydrates. Refined, process carbs usually come in a box or a bag. Shoot for starches that contain at least 3 grams of fiber per serving.

4. Consume 25 to 35 grams of fiber per day. Since the average diet contains only 14 grams of fiber, adding foods that are fiber-rich is a must. Fiber helps satisfy hunger pangs, as well as control insulin and blood sugar levels, which, when elevated, tend to promote fat storage.

5. Eat some type of lean protein at each meal. Protein helps satisfy hunger and provides the necessary building blocks to maintain lean body mass while you lose body fat. And protein provides high a Thermic Effect, which burns calories – I'll talk more in depth about this later.

6. Consume adequate amounts of healthy-fat foods, such as olive oil, walnuts, almonds, Omega-3

fortified eggs or other Omega-3 products. Healthy fats are great antioxidants, and they help with brain function and many other of the body's essentials processes. Essential Fatty Acids (EFA) also help prevent certain diseases.

7. Get 10 servings of fruits and vegetables a day to meet your micronutrient needs. Vegetables contain a good amount of fiber and help control your appetite.

8. Follow a plan. Map out your meals every day and follow them. If you follow your plan every day for 3 weeks, you will eventually form habits that become part of your daily routine. Good habits, like bad ones, are formed by doing something over and over again.

9. Include what I call *"Superfoods"* in your meal plan on a daily basis. These foods include lean meat, salmon, low-fat plain yogurt, tomatoes, spinach, mixed berries, whole oats, mixed nuts, olive oil, flax seeds (or flax meal), green tea and various beans. Later, we will discuss all my *Superfood* recommendations.

10. **EXERCISE!** It's possible for some people to lose weight by just following a nutrition plan alone. But it takes much longer than if you combine good nutrition with exercise. Go back to the section above on exercise for tips on what type of exercise to do, and how often.

11. Record what you eat and drink. You'd be amazed at what you consume without even realizing it. Keeping a food log is critical to your success. If changes aren't happening like you had hoped, the answer as to why usually lies in your food journal.

12. Follow the 90% rule. Following your plan 90% of the time is enough to succeed with weight loss. Lose the all-or-nothing attitude and take one day at a time. Reflect on your day before you go to bed at night. Instead of getting down on yourself because you weren't perfect that day, set goals to do better tomorrow.

Chapter 3:

Yes, It's True: You Are What You Eat

Now that you're becoming aware of how the proper foods play an important role in your weight loss success, let's take it a step further. In this chapter, you'll discover more about how and why selecting certain foods helps you dramatically reduce your body fat, once and for all!

Protein

As I've said already, protein is one of the keys to losing weight. Not only does it provide the amino acids needed to boost muscle growth, it also helps in the prevention of muscle breakdown.

Another key thing protein does is stimulate a hormone called glucagon. Carbohydrates stimulate insulin, which prevents the body from releasing stored fat to be used for energy. Protein and glucagon have the opposite effect - they help the *release* of stored body fat.

Increased protein consumption allows you to feel fuller quicker than if you eat other types of foods. The result?

You're less likely to overeat.

Finally, in addition to increasing your metabolic rate, protein is considered a caloric expensive nutrient, meaning it requires more energy to digest and break down than other nutrients.

Below are some good sources of lean protein.

- Chicken breast
- Turkey breast
- Ground turkey
- Ham
- Lean ground beef
- Tuna (packed in water)
- Kidney beans
- Non-fat cottage cheese
- Skim milk
- Egg
- Yogurt (low fat)
- Egg whites
- Fish

Carbohydrates

Carbohydrates affect the body in many ways. Different carbohydrates affect insulin levels, which affect how your body utilizes and stores this nutrient. There is much discussion on how the "glycemic index" of foods affects insulin levels and the utilization of carbohydrates.

Foods that are high on the glycemic index (also known as quick-digesting carbohydrates) generate a high insulin response, which causes your body to store calories for energy or as fat. The objective is to eat foods that reduce that insulin spike. High insulin levels also inhibit the release of stored fat cells to be used for energy. Carbohydrates that have high fiber content (like whole grains) tend to cause a lower rise in insulin levels, so choose these carb sources whenever possible.

Low-glycemic index foods (such as vegetables) also tend to have a better nutritional value and more fiber. Plus, they help you feel fuller at meals, maintain better insulin sensitivity and contribute to fat loss.

Below are the carbohydrates you should be choosing most often to achieve the goal of lower glycemic consumption and reduced insulin response.

- **Select Most Often**

Amaranth	Barley
Beans	Brown rice
Buckwheat	Oatmeal
Whole rye	Wholegrain bread
Whole-wheat crackers	Whole-wheat pasta
Whole-wheat tortillas	Wild rice

- **Select Moderately**

Cornbread	Corn tortillas
Couscous	Crackers
Flour tortillas	Noodles
Spaghetti	Macaroni
Most breakfast cereals	Pretzels
White bread	White buns, rolls
White rice	

Fat

There are good fats and bad fats. Science tells us we need fat in our diet to function properly. It's the *type* of fat that makes the difference. The best approach is to plan your diet so it contains 1/3 of each type of fat: monounsaturated, polyunsaturated and saturated. Monounsaturated and polyunsaturated fats are found in fish, nuts and oils. These are the fats that fall into the "Select Most Often" and "Select Moderately" lists (see below). Saturated fats are found in the "Select Least Often" category – remember, you want to limit this type of fat in your diet.

Unfortunately, today's poor quality diets and processed foods create deficiencies in 2 very important fats: DHA and EPA, otherwise known as Essential Fatty Acids.

Scientific research shows that consuming sufficient quantities of DHA and EPA helps prevent cancer, heart disease, depression and other diseases.

Essential Fatty Acids (EFA) such as DHA and EPA are crucial for normal health and metabolism. EFA cannot be manufactured in the body, so we must get it through our diet. You've probably heard of 2 types of EFA: Omega 6 fat and Omega 3 fat. Most people eat too much Omega 6 fat and not enough Omega 3 fat. In fact, most people's diets consist of a ratio of 20:1 Omega 6 to Omega 3 fats.

This is a problem because too much Omega 6 fat promotes the production of inflammation-causing chemicals in the body. Omega 3's, on the other hand, encourage the production of inflammation-fighting chemicals. Omega 6 fats are found in foods such as corn, soy, canola and sunflower oil, which are used in store-bought, processed foods. We need more Omega 3 fats, such as flaxseed oil, fish, fish oil, extra virgin olive oil and avocados.

Some scientists believe this unbalanced ratio of Omega 6 fat and Omega 3 fat is contributing to heart disease, cancer and obesity. This is why I recommend a high quality fish oil supplement, along with consuming high quality "good" fats (see the list below). This not only decreases your risk for disease, it improves your overall quality of life.

- **Select Most Often**

Avocado	Flax oil
Fish oil	Olive oil
Olives	Mixed nuts
Sunflower oil	

- **Select Moderately**

Egg yolks	Margarine
Vegetable oil	

- **Select Least Often**

Animal fat	Butter
Cream	Fried foods
Ice cream	Sour cream
Whole-fat dairy products	

Strategies for Limiting Fat Intake

Here are some strategies for reducing intake of unhealthy dietary fat.

- Choose nonfat, low-fat or reduced-fat dressings.

- Select broth-based soups instead of cream-based soups.
- Add alternative seasonings or foods when cooking. Examples: onions, garlic, mushrooms, chicken stock, peppers, salsa, horseradish, teriyaki sauce, soy sauce, herbs and spices.
- Use cooking sprays instead of butter, margarine or vegetable oil when cooking. When a recipe calls for oil, opt for olive oil.

Is Fiber a Super-Nutrient?

Fiber. It's been touted as a way to lower cholesterol, reduce the risk of heart disease, help you to lose weight … is fiber some sort of super-nutrient? Pretty much.

Here are the facts.

1. Fiber is considered useful for treating obesity, heart disease and diabetes.

2. The USDA suggests eating 20 to 35 grams of dietary fiber per day (sadly, the average America only gets 12 to 15 grams). Consuming the recommended amount of fiber may lower cholesterol, control blood sugars and reduce obesity.

3. Studies show that consuming a fiber-rich diet may decrease the number of overall calories you eat throughout the day. In as little as 4 months, subjects who

increased their fiber intake lost an average of 5 pounds - with no dieting.

4. Including 5 to 6 servings of fruits and vegetables - along with 4 to 8 servings of nutrient-dense wholegrain starches - ensures you benefit from 20 to 35 grams of fiber per day.

5. Fiber slows the digestion process, which helps control food cravings and blood sugars (very important for weight loss and how the body stores fat). Fiber also improves the absorption of minerals and other nutrients during digestion.

6. Look for foods that provide at least 2 to 3 grams of fiber per serving. These are considered good sources of fiber.

7. General guidelines for increasing your fiber intake: Eat more fruits, vegetables, beans and nuts. Go for raw, unpeeled fruits and vegetables. Use wholegrain breads and cereals instead of refined products. Increase your fluid intake.

The table below shows the top 15 sources of high-fiber foods. These foods are also highly recommended for weight loss and healthy eating because they provide nutrition and make you feel full.

Food	Dietary Fiber (grams)	Calories
Navy beans, cooked ½ cup	9.5	128
Bran (ready-to-eat cereal 100%) ½ cup	8.8	78
Kidney beans ½ cup	8.2	109
Split peas (cooked) ½ cup	8.1	116
Lentils (cooked) ½ cup	7.8	115
Black beans (cooked) ½ cup	7.5	114
Pinto beans (cooked) ½ cup	7.7	122
Lima beans (cooked) ½ cup	6.6	108
Artichoke (cooked) 1	6.5	60
White beans ½ cup	6.3	154

Chickpeas (cooked) ½ cup	6.2	135
Crackers, rye 2 wafers	5.0	74
Sweet potato with peel 1	4.8	131
Green peas (cooked) ½ cup	4.4	67
Mixed vegetables (cooked) ½ cup	4.0	59

TIP

Did you know that water is a natural appetite suppressant? Drink 8 to 12 oz. of water about 20 minutes before you eat a meal. This helps control hunger and forces you to eat less food simply because you feel more full.

Water

Water is involved in every function of the body, so if you don't consume enough of it your body won't run efficiently (yes, that means a slower metabolism). When you're properly hydrated, your body is more efficient at burning calories.

Water helps you lose weight in another way, too. You see, when someone's dehydrated, they might mistake that feeling for hunger. Some studies show that thirst and hunger are triggered together, so you may reach for food when all you need is a glass of water.

In general, you should drink about 1 oz. of water for every 1.5 to 2 lbs of bodyweight. For most people, this amounts to 10 to 18 cups of water a day. Notice that this is much higher than the standard 8 glasses a day we hear so much about!

To make sure you get your daily dose of water, make it part of your everyday routine. For example:

- Take a bottle of water with you in the car
- Keep a water bottle at your office desk
- Drink a glass of water at every coffee break and at lunchtime
- Bring water with you into a meeting
- Drink a bottle of water on your way home from work
- Have a glass of water at arm's reach while you make dinner
- Serve water at the dinner table (in addition to whatever else you drink)

Not All Calories Are Created Equal

The kind of food you put in your mouth, and when you eat it, may determine the amount of calories you burn. The simple fact is, not all calories are created equal.

Every time you eat food, a reaction takes place called the "Thermic Effect of Food (TEF)." TEF is the cost of energy your body burns to break down and digest food to make it a usable energy source. Simply put, it's the calories you burn during digestion. TEF lasts from 1 to 4 hours after you eat and makes up around 10% of your total calorie expenditure every day.

You can boost TEF by eating foods that have a higher TEF effect. So what are they? Well, researchers have determined that protein, carbohydrates and fat have different TEF ratios. Here's how it breaks down:

Protein: 25 to 30% TEF

Carbohydrates: 7% TEF

Fat: 3% TEF

For example, if you ate 100 calories of only protein, your body would use 25 to 30 calories to digest and utilize that protein. If you ate 100 calories of pure carbohydrates, your body would use 7 calories to digest and utilize that carbohydrate. And fat? Three measly calories. Your body uses just 3 calories to digest 100 calories of fat.

So there you have it - protein has a significantly higher TEF compared to carbohydrate or fat. You may eat the same number of calories for protein, carbohydrates and fat, but the result is less overall calories for the protein source.

The TEF of various foods is important for weight loss. Science tells us that eating a higher proportion of protein burns more calories and raises your metabolism (plus, it makes you feel fuller, so you eat less).

The importance of *what* we eat is supported by science. *When* we eat is also significant, scientists say. Next, let's look at how the timing of meals and snacks can influence certain hormones responsible for muscle growth, fat burning and other necessary physical functions

Chapter 4:

Accelerating Your Results

I briefly talked earlier in this book on the importance of vegetables and fruit in your diet and how they counteract the acidity of your protein intake. To recap that part real quick here is what I discussed. I will then go into further detail and how you can accelerate the work you put in the gym.

"A high protein diet, which is an essential part of building muscle, but protein actually puts your body into an acidic state. Too much acidity can lead to a host of various health issues. To counter this your body uses alkaline foods (plant foods and greens). If you are not eating enough alkaline foods though your body will pull glutamine and other vital nutrients right out of your muscle.

It will break down your muscle to free up your glutamine. Obviously this is something none of us want or else we wouldn't be going to the gym to build new muscle. By consuming plenty of vegetables each and every day will allow you to still consume plenty of lean protein for muscle building, but keep your body pH balanced for optimal muscle growth."

Now that we have the overall understanding of why a pH balanced body is so important to your results here is how you accelerate your muscle building results.

If you struggle with types of gains that others see or your own gains are just slow it can boil down to what is in your body and what you are not putting into your body. Adding more sets, working out harder or longer isn't going to solve this.

Not consuming the proper nutrients can impact your immune system, digestive system and your metabolism. This is so impactful that you can plateau regardless of how much time you put in the gym.

When you are all about building new muscle so many people focus just on the macro-nutrients such as protein and carbs. It is the micronutrients though that optimize your body to build new muscle. Those micronutrients come from fruits and vegetables.

Think about this for second.

When you think of your immune system do you associate it with not getting sick or not getting a cold?

Did you know that all that strength training you do and muscle building activates your immune response?

Your immune system is what repairs all those micro tears you created in your muscles. So if your immune system isn't strong enough or doesn't have enough micronutrients then it can't repair your muscles. Not too mention you are now at a higher risk for getting an infection also.

Free radicals start to consume your body and your body has to focus on fighting off other health issues instead of repairing your muscle before you get back to the gym.

Oh, did I mention the internal inflammation that is building and the chronic inflammation that can result if you don't boost your immune system. Inflammation slows your muscle recovery and can lead to overtraining.

The Solution: Nutrient Extraction

In this program I have laid out how you can get a good amount of vegetables and fruit into your nutrition program, but there is a way to speed up absorption of your micronutrients and increase the amount of these micronutrients and it is juicing.

You can conquer these obstacles to accelerated muscle growth and massive gains with this simple way of consuming higher bioavailable micronutrients, fruits and vegetables.

The basic purpose is to reset your digestive system by cleansing it. When you are able to absorb nutrients faster and more efficiently your immune system is now freed up to repair your muscle tissue from the workouts.

You will have fewer free radicals floating around in the body with fewer bouts of illness and more importantly less inflammation. You will notice less aches, pains and even less cramping after a workout.

Your metabolism will speed significantly getting rid of your excess body fat. You will find that with less inflammation, optimized immune system and faster metabolism you will be able to eat more food and still lose body fat in a shorter amount of time.

So what do you have to do to get all these benefits. You can buy a juicer or you can purchase a high powered blender such as a Vitamix or Ninja Blender. Timing is important to get the most benefit.

Here are some guidelines to follow:

First thing in the morning you should consume a green drink. This will jumpstart your metabolism and give you an energy boost to start your day.

Then drink a 2nd drink in the afternoon. The afternoon drink can be a fruit based drink.

Your goal is 2 drinks a day to maximize the cleansing of your system and optimizing your body for muscle building. If you want more than 2 that is perfectly fine.

Appendix C at the end of this book provides some recipes for you to get started.

Chapter 5:

Nutrient Timing Hacks: Rapid Fat Loss to Achieve That Lean Body

When it comes to rapid fat loss many individuals will create expectations that they just can't stick to or follow. All this does is set you up for failure. Instead you can still create rapid fat loss, but do so with smaller expectations. You will start to compound and build on these expectations and that creates your rapid fat loss.

It is all about looking the the big Goal or Objective and then breaking it down into smaller bit size chunks. For example if you wanted to save $500 to buy a TV. Instead of thinking about how to come up with all $500 at once you would break it down into small achievable goals.

Such as these:

I am going to bring my lunch to work every day instead of eating out. Weekly savings: $37.

I am going to use coupons when I go grocery shopping. Weekly savings: $9

I am going to stick to the essentials for groceries and take advantage of only sale items. Weekly savings: $35

Now you see in just a few short weeks or 1 month you can have that $500 for the TV because you accomplished many small achievable goals.

Consistency in working toward your goals is a key to long term success.

Here Is How You Can Achieve Rapid Fat Loss With Proper Food Timing

One of the keys to improving your metabolism and increasing your TEF during the day is to eat every 2 to 3 hours, including consuming lean protein with each meal or snack.

Researchers from Queen's Medical Centre in the United Kingdom reported that subjects who ate meals at irregular times showed significantly lower TEF than those who ate at regular times – i.e., every 2 to 3 hours during the waking day. Bottom line: Eating regular meals that consist of lean protein turns your metabolism into a calorie-burning furnace all day long. More calories burned equals more fat loss.

However, the timing of when you consume certain *types* of calories is also important to successful fat loss. Your body metabolizes and utilizes carbohydrates best in the morning, after you wake up (and after you work out, which I'll get to in a moment).

Therefore, the morning is the ideal time to consume quick-digesting carbohydrates (also known as high-glycemic carbs) versus slower-digesting ones, such as whole grains, vegetables and fruit carbohydrates. The reason your body uses calories best in the morning is because you've been fasting all night as you sleep. This elevates cortisol levels. While some cortisol is important for the body, levels that are too high encourage fat storage and are detrimental to muscle growth. Not what we want.

Cortisol levels are also higher after a workout. To control cortisol levels in the morning or after exercise, your goal is to elevate insulin levels, which suppress cortisol levels. After workouts, we are more sensitive to insulin, which allows the body to use fast-digesting carbohydrates as energy rather than storing them as fat. The insulin levels also help with other aspects of recovering from exercise, so you can give it your all during every workout.

How does all this facilitate fat loss? It has to do with nutrient timing. And, believe it or not, sugar.

Some people say all sugar is bad and should be avoided at all costs. Others recommend eating fruits and vegetables (which contain natural sugars). Which is it?

The fear about sugar is that it increases insulin levels, which promotes fat storage and decreases fat loss. This is true - to an extent. However, most people forget that there are many nutrients and mechanisms that help control insulin levels, such as fiber and the carbohydrates recommended in this book.

In the previous chapter, I advised you to avoid eating too many high-glycemic (or quick-digesting) carbohydrates. However, for reasons I described in this chapter, you may eat them - in moderation, of course – first thing in the morning.

And there's another exception: Research shows that consuming quick-digesting carbohydrates along with protein after a workout benefits your body's ability to recover from exercise and also increases fat oxidation (fat your body burns for energy).

Bottom line: Don't be afraid to eat high-glycemic, or quick-digesting, carbohydrates at breakfast or after your workouts – as long as you also include a good source of lean protein. Doing so will help you achieve your weight-loss goals.

Carb Timing

This part I won't elaborate on because Chapter 1 of this book covers all this and is the basis of Flexible Carb-Cycling. If you need a review go back to Chapter 1, but understand that this is the essence of nutrient timing and why it is so effective for rapid fat loss.

How to Eat Before Bed:

I get this question asked quite a lot and it is Do I need to or should I be eating before I go to bed?

The answer is "It depends". Most individuals will benefit from eating lean protein late at night. The reason is a few things. It keeps you from craving late night unhealthy sugary snacks. It provides some essential amino acids and healthy calories to help your body repair itself while you sleep. Most of your recovery occurs while you sleep so you want to make sure you have the necessary nutrients to provide your body the building blocks to repair itself.

Some good lean protein examples are cottage cheese, protein powder, or greek yogurt.

One trick that I use is I take greek yogurt and mix in a slow digesting protein powder called casein. Essentially I make chocolate pudding this way. ☺

Always Eat Carbs with Protein

All carbs have an impact on your blood sugars and insulin response. This creates a fat storing environment you want to avoid. An easy way to do this is to combine your carbs with some type of lean protein.

Consuming lean protein at every meal will allow your body to stay at a steady level of insulin response and create a muscle preserving fat burning level. The protein also provides essential amino acids to build new lean muscle and repair muscle damage.

The thermic effect of including protein at every meal will speed up your metabolism as it requires more calories to digest and utilize protein. It is more metabolically active. It will also help you keep cravings to a minimum when you include protein with carbs.

Use Shirataki noodles on Low Carb Days and Even No Carb Days

If you have never heard of Shirataki noodles you are missing out on a very low calorie noodle.

How is that possible?

Aren't noodles carbohydrates and didn't I just read that too many carbs are bad?

This noodle is different....

It is a noodle that is made of a soluble fiber called Glucomannan. Here is a bulleted list derived from www.Konjacfoods.com

Shirataki noodles ....

- are naturally water soluble fiber with no fat, sugar, starch, or protein.
- contain zero net carbohydrates and zero calories.
- are wheat and gluten free.
- Pure Vegetable
- can be stored in the room temperature for about one year. Don't need refrigeration
- JAS (Japan Agricultural Standard) Cetified Organic

- are translucent and gelatinous, with no flavor of their own - they easily absorb the dominant flavors of any soup or dish.
- are instant and come in a variety of styles and shapes - you can simply toss salsa with Konjac instant pasta for a quick meal

It is pretty amazing how easily these noodles absorb whatever flavorings you add to your recipe or dish. They are so versatile they can be eaten cold or hot.

Check out www.Konjacfoods.com and they have hundreds of recipes to choose from using Shirataki noodles.

Chapter 6:

Building a Better Meal Plan

We went over your calorie needs during the first 30 days, but I'd like to discuss it again here as a review. On the Flexible Carb-Cycling Diet, you determined your calorie needs. But you only used this number as a reference. You didn't count calories at every meal or every day.

Earlier in this book, I showed you the formula for determining your body's daily calorie needs.

Converting Calories to Food Exchanges

There's another way to plan your meals besides counting calories – with something called food exchanges. Why convert calories to exchanges? Because your life is too busy to count calories all day long. Tallying up calories is not an efficient way to eat healthfully day in and day out. Plus, it's time-consuming and a bit neurotic to track every last calorie you eat.

Look, in the grand scheme of eating well, it doesn't matter if an apple amounts to 68 calories or 74 calories.

Does it? What counts is the healthy choices you make each day. Many people lose weight without ever counting a single calorie.

So why did I have you calculate that formula for your daily caloric needs? I want you to have a baseline of calories, so you can determine your food exchanges.

What Are Food Exchanges?

A "food exchange" is a fancy way of describing something you're already familiar with: serving sizes! Here's how it works: As you may know, there are 6 main food categories.

1. Dairy
2. Vegetable
3. Fruit
4. Starch
5. Protein
6. Fat

Each of these categories has a calorie guideline that equals **1 serving of food** for that category. Some categories also have subcategories (such as with Dairy and Protein below). For example:

Dairy:

Low fat: 1 serving = 90 calories
Reduced fat: 1 serving = 120 calories
Whole-milk products: 1 serving = 150 calories

Vegetable: 1 serving = 25 calories

Fruit: 1 serving = 60 calories

Starch: (bread, cereal, rice, pastas): 1 serving = 80 calories

Protein:

Lean protein and meat substitutes (0 to 3 grams of fat): 1 serving = 35 to 55 calories, respectively

Medium-fat protein and meat substitutes: 1 serving = 75 calories

High-fat protein and meat substitutes: 1 serving = 100 calories

Fat: 1 serving = 45 calories

Appendix A in this book explains what foods equal 1 serving for each of the above groups. The information there is designed to help you meet your daily serving requirements with foods you enjoy. For example, 1 oz. of plain chicken breast equals 1 serving of protein. But you may choose a 2-oz. chicken breast flavored with low-calorie marinade. That equals 2 servings of protein. You will also be able to dine at a restaurant or friend's place and still determine how many calories are on your plate.

How to Convert Calories to Food Exchanges

Now it's time to convert your calorie needs to exchanges. I will explain how to do this manually, but you can also refer to the exchange lists for different calorie counts in Appendix B.

To manually convert calories to servings sizes, determine your proper nutrient ratio. So, if you've reached your weight loss goals and want to maintain your new, thin body, your nutrient ratio should be around 45% carbohydrates, 35% protein and 20% fat.

For example, let's say your calorie needs are 1,850 calories per day. You would do the following calculations:

1,850 x 45% (carbs) = 832 calories

1,850 x 35% (protein) = 647 calories

1,850 x 20% (fat) = 370 calories

These are the calories you need to eat from each nutrient ratio.

Carbohydrates: 832 calories

Protein: 647 calories

Fat: 370 calories

Now it gets a bit trickier because you have to know how many grams of these nutrients are in each exchange category. Don't worry, I'm not going to give you more formulas to work out. Simply go to Appendix B and find the allotted number of calories you should be eating in a day (e.g., 1,800, 2,000, 2,200, etc.).

The numbers in Appendix B are in 100-calorie increments. Round up if your calorie level falls above the halfway mark (e.g., 2,060 = 2,100); round down for calorie levels below the halfway mark (e.g., 2, 040 = 2,000).

An example of how the chart in Appendix B works.

Calories: 1,850 (round up to 1,900)
Ratio: 45/35/20
Dairy: 4
Vegetable: 8
Fruit: 4
Starch: 4
Protein: 11
Fat: 5

TIP

If you exercise 4 to 5 times per week, you need higher carbs. If you're less active or not active at all, you need lower carbs. Modify the exchanges to fit your lifestyle (and work toward creating an active lifestyle for yourself).

Laying Out Your Exchanges

Laying out the 45/35/20 ratio of exchanges is already done for you. Just go to Appendix B and follow the suggested layout of how you should eat throughout the day.

Notice the exchanges are spread out so you eat some type of protein and vegetable at every meal whenever possible. This accomplishes 2 things: 1) you get a variety of nutrients throughout the day, and 2) you efficiently fuel your body to maximize your metabolism.

You don't have to follow the layout in Appendix B exactly. You can create your own plan however you'd like. Just remember to spread your exchanges out as evenly as possible throughout the day.

How to Build Your Meals

Remember when your parents doled out the proper portions of food on your plate, then told you to finish everything? This practice was fine when dinner plates were smaller and the entire surface wasn't covered with food.

Dinner plates today are often much larger than they used to be – yet we still fill the entire plate with food! One key way you can maintain a healthy weight is by controlling portion sizes.

Research has shown that people often underestimate how many daily calories they consume by as much as 25%. Until now, I've been explaining a lot about the right kinds of foods to eat for weight loss and maintenance. However, eating the right *amount* of food at each meal is just as important.

Proper portion sizes might be smaller than you realize.

Estimating portion size is easy once you know what a proper portion size looks like. Use the portion chart shown below to help give you an idea of typical serving sizes.

Cheese - 1 ounce/28 grams of cheese = 4 dice

Fruit - 1 fruit serving = baseball

Vegetables - ½ cup/120 ml = ½ a baseball

Pasta/rice – ½ cup/120 ml = ½ a baseball

Fish/meat – 1 serving of cooked

   meat, fish or poultry = deck of cards

Peanut butter - 2 tablespoons/30 ml of

   peanut butter = large marshmallow

Dairy- 1 cup/240 ml of milk, yogurt = a fist

Butter – 1 teaspoon/5 ml = pat of butter

Bread – 1 serving of carbohydrate = 1 slice

Salad dressing – 2 tablespoons/30 ml = standard ice cube

Potato – ½ a potato = ½ a baseball

When you make your plate for each meal, choose, for example, 1 protein serving, 1 starch/carbohydrate serving and 2 servings of vegetables and/or a fruit. Using a portion control chart like the one above shows you there should be plenty of empty space on your plate! Overloading your plate leads to overeating.

To properly build a meal, write down your total daily servings, including how many of those servings you should have at each meal. Record the results on a piece of paper or excel spreadsheet. Now go to Appendix A and choose foods of the appropriate serving sizes. Create your meal plans for multiple days in advance to help keep you compliant with your new approach to eating.

TIP

You can combine servings at one meal. For example, if dinner calls for 5 oz. of protein, you can have a 5 oz. chicken breast instead of breaking it up into 5 separate servings of protein.

Foods to Select Most Often

Below is a list of foods that I consider staples in any meal plan. They're nutrient-dense, good for your metabolism and make you feel full. Try to incorporate a variety of these foods into your daily meals.

Lean Protein Sources:

- Chicken or turkey (white meat)
- Tuna fish (canned, in water)
- Lean beef
- Egg whites
- Non-fat cottage cheese

- Fish like shark, salmon, flounder (farmed often have the least contaminants)
- Shellfish

"Medium-Fat" Protein Sources:

- Chicken or turkey (dark meat)
- Whole eggs
- Cottage cheese (2% or whole)
- Steaks (moderate-fat cuts, 20 to 25% fat)
- Other meats (moderate fat, 20 to 25% fat)
- Mozzarella cheese (nonfat or skim)

Vegetables:

- Broccoli
- Salad (lettuce, romaine lettuce, etc.); use nonfat salad dressing
- Cabbage
- Green beans
- Spinach
- Zucchini
- Squash
- Red or green pepper
- Asparagus
- Carrots
- Tomatoes
- Cauliflower
- Mushrooms

- Artichoke hearts

Carbohydrates:

- Sweet potatoes or yams
- Brown rice
- Corn
- Peas
- Legumes (chickpeas, lima beans, lentils, dry beans)
- High-fiber cereals (All Bran, Fiber One, Grape Nuts, Cracklin' Oat Bran, Shredded Wheat)
- Oats and oatmeal (not instant oatmeal)
- Black beans
- 100% Wholegrain pasta (Eden, Hodgson Mill, Purity Foods)
- 100% Wholegrain bread (Pepperidge Farm, Nature's Path, Nature's Own, Earth Grains)

High-Fiber Fruits:

- Raspberries
- Strawberries
- Blackberries
- Apples
- Pears
- Prunes
- Oranges

Eating Out: Is It Possible?

What choices do you make when you eat at a restaurant? Can you ever eat out again?

Yes, you can eat out. Many restaurants now have lean or low-calorie meals to accommodate healthy eaters like you. Choose a dish from the restaurant's low-calorie menu, and follow my guidelines for dining out:

- Find fast-food restaurants that grill their meats rather than fry them.
- Choose grilled chicken over a double-patty melt.
- Keep sandwiches plain. Add your own condiments like mustard. Steer clear of a restaurant's special sauces and cheeses.
- Choose a baked potato or beans instead of fries and coleslaw.
- Fill your plate with plenty of vegetables.
- Order salad with dressing on the side; pick oil-and-vinegar dressings to boost your intake of Omega 3 fatty acids.
- Drink water (not soda) to satisfy thirst and reduce calories.

7 Specific Superfoods to Include in Your Diet Every Day

I have a list of superfoods that I like to include in every client's meal plan. These foods are very nutrient-dense and contain many disease-fighting properties. Here, I share my favorite superfoods with you. Please make them part of your own meal plan.

1. Fruit

The following fruits are high in antioxidants to help prevent disease. They also contain flavonoids that help with eyesight and coordination. The dark-colored fruits also provide fiber and boost your immune system.

Fruits I especially recommend:

- Raspberries
- Blueberries
- Blackberries
- Guava (great source of lycopene)
- Goji berries
- Dried plums

2. Nuts

Nuts are a great source of fiber, vitamin B6, niacin, magnesium, healthy monounsaturated fats, protein and more. Nuts help lower LDL (bad) cholesterol and may help maintain healthy blood vessels, as well.

Nuts I especially recommend:

- Almonds
- Walnuts
- Cashews
- Brazil nuts
- Hazelnuts

3. Beans/Lentils

Beans are a great source of protein and fiber – and they're low in calories. Beans help stabilize blood sugars and provide isoflavones, which help prevent certain forms of cancers and heart disease.

Beans I especially recommend:

- Legumes (chickpeas, lima beans, lentils, dry beans)
- Black beans
- Red beans

4. Oils

Oils - particularly Extra Virgin Olive Oil - are examples of heart-healthy fat that helps lower LDL (bad) cholesterol. Oils contain antioxidant and anti-inflammatory properties, as well. And they help control food cravings.

Oils I especially recommend:

- Extra Virgin Olive Oil
- Fish oil

5. Fish

Fish contains the potent Omega 3 fatty acid, which helps your body store less fat and convert fat to energy. Fish is a great anti-inflammatory and a wonderful "brain food." The ADA recommends 1.5 to 3 grams of Omega 3 fat a day. One serving of the choices below provides almost 4 grams of Omega 3 fat.

Fish I especially recommend:

- Salmon
- Tuna
- Mackerel

6. Vegetables

A variety of color is key when selecting vegetables. For example, orange carrots are a great source of beta carotene, which can reduce the risk of cancer. Red tomatoes contain lycopene, another powerful antioxidant for reducing the risk of cancer. Dark green, leafy vegetables, such as spinach, contain carotenoids that improve your immune system and are full of vitamins and minerals. Broccoli, cauliflower, kale and other cruciferous vegetables contain cancer-fighting properties.

Vegetables I especially recommend:

- Carrots
- Tomatoes
- Broccoli
- Kale
- Spinach
- Cauliflower
- Beets
- Cabbage
- Swiss chard
- Purslane (used as a salad green or herb)

7. Green Tea

Not only is non-caffeinated fluid good for you, research shows that green tea may be one of the best disease-fighting beverages you can consume. It's very high in antioxidants and has cancer-fighting properties. Green tea may actually inhibit the growth of cancer cells, according to research. Other research shows it reduces overall cholesterol levels and increases the ratio of HDL (good) cholesterol to LDL (bad) cholesterol.

Here are just some of the ailments that drinking green tea helps:

- cancer
- rheumatoid arthritis
- high cholesterol levels
- cardiovascular disease
- infection
- impaired immune function

Finally, research suggests that drinking green tea also benefits those who want to lose weight. Subjects who consumed caffeine plus green tea extract burned more calories than those who consumed caffeine or a placebo. More studies are needed to determine if this evidence is valid, but so far it looks encouraging.

Chapter 7:

Shopping & Cooking Made Easy

You must learn the right way to navigate through a grocery store – yes, it's probably different from how you do it now. You see, a grocery store's strategy is to funnel you into the center of the store where all the sales and endcap special items are located. Generally, this is also where the unhealthiest foods are stocked. Next time you're at the grocery store, notice that the sales items are at the end of each aisle. This design is meant to keep enticing you with specials, so you start putting these products in your cart. It's not that grocery stores want you to pass up all the healthy foods. It's just that there are so many more unhealthy products that need to be sold.

Strategies for Buying the Right Foods

I just explained the grocery store's strategy for getting you to buy food. What's yours? Well, your first step should be to have a plan, one you implement before you set foot in the store. Lay out your meal plans for the week. Determine what foods you need, and how much.

Second, do not go to the store while you are hungry. Ever notice that when you're hungry every food looks appealing? Shop after a meal so your hunger pangs don't persuade you to buy foods you don't need.

Third, know the route to take once you enter the store. This step is pretty much taken care of if you created your meal plans correctly. Generally, the healthiest foods are stocked around the perimeter of the grocery store. This is where you find fruits, vegetables, meats, fish and dairy. Sure, there are also healthy foods in the middle of the store, but most of the healthiest foods are around the perimeter.

TIP

To save money on your grocery bill, look for generic or store-brand products. These products are almost always cheaper, and they generally have the exact same ingredients as the bigger brand-name products.

Once you have completed your shopping, here are some ways to save time on food preparation throughout the week.

- Chop your vegetables twice a week. Chop up the first half of your vegetables for the week and store them in Ziploc bags or Tupperware-type containers. Then mid-week, chop up the remaining vegetables for the week.

- Cook your protein (meats) for the first half of the week, then again mid-week for the second half of the week.

- Cook your fiber-rich starches at the beginning of the week. Wild rice, whole oats, etc., can be cooked ahead of time, then stored to eat throughout the week.

- Keep everything in Tupperware-type containers, so when you are ready to make a meal, you have all the preparation complete – all you have to do is assemble your meal and enjoy.

Chapter 8:

There's No Magic Pill, But …

There are hundreds, if not thousands, of nutritional supplements on the shelves today. Some are good, and some are, frankly, garbage. How are you to determine what's what, and if you should even be taking supplements?

Well, I'm here to advise you that there are supplements you should be taking. I've done the research for you, so you'll know which brand to get, what you should take, and why.

I've seen more awful supplements than I've seen good ones. Based on this experience, I know how to weed out the bad products in favor of good ones. And I have my finger on the pulse of research that shows what's most effective in this area.

In this chapter, I share with you which supplements are most effective for helping you lose weight. So without further ado …

1. One of the largest to date human studies conducted on a finished weight loss formula.

It seems like every month a new weight loss supplement is being touted as a shortcut or fat loss "cure." There's no doubt you're familiar with nutritional supplement claims of boosting your metabolism or blasting fat away—the unfortunate truth is that many of these claims are unsupported hype. But some exciting new scientific discoveries could change all that. Recently the fat-fighting supplement raspberry ketones have caused quite a stir in the weight loss industry. It's got people on forums, personal trainers and even medical TV personalities singing its praises.

Berries have long been regarded as a superfood providing many health-boosting benefits. They are powerful antioxidants, promote brain health and cognition, support a healthy cardiovascular system and help with blood sugar management, plus they have anti-inflammatory properties. Now research is suggesting that a component of the raspberry known as raspberry ketones may aid in weight loss.

In a supplement form you're able to consume a concentrated enough dosage of raspberry ketones for the weight loss and fat-burning benefits.

#1—Speeding Up Your Metabolism

Your metabolism is the rate at which your body uses calories. At the end of the day if you've used more calories than you've consumed you will lose weight.

Traditionally we would think that the only way to use more calories is to exercise, but, as research is now showing, it's possible to actually increase the body's metabolism naturally with a supplement like raspberry ketones. In essence, by using raspberry ketones and speeding up your metabolism, you burn more calories without any additional exercise.

#2—Accelerating Fat Burning

On top of speeding up your metabolism, raspberry ketones also increase the efficiency of the body's ability to use or burn fat as a fuel source. This happens through a function called lipolysis, which breaks down the fat into more accessible energy so the body can actually utilize it. Normally, burning fat requires certain conditions and processes to utilize it. Raspberry ketones are able to cause fat cells to get broken down more effectively, therefore helping the body to use the fat as fuel. The end result is essentially "burning fat" at a higher and faster rate. Remember we spoke earlier about how burning the fat from fat cells will actually shrink the fat cells and result in those areas of your body looking thinner and slimmer.

#3—Regulates Fat-Burning Protein

Lastly, raspberry ketones have been shown to regulate an integral protein for weight loss called adiponectin. Adiponectin plays a pivotal role in many functions related to weight loss, including metabolic processes, glucose regulation and the breakdown of fat for energy. Regulating and having optimal functioning of such an important weight loss protein such as adiponectin can play a vital part in the fat reduction of individuals who struggle to lose weight or have reached a plateau with their weight loss efforts. If these underlying processes inside the body that relate to weight loss are not in order, it can literally be like fighting an uphill battle as the body is not functioning properly and not in an optimal state to lose weight.

Not only is this nutrient in this clinically studied formula, but there are others that make this fomula one of the most potent weight loss supplements on the market. Oh and did I forget to mention that this study has been published and is one of the safest weight loss formulas on the market to date.

You can learn more about this clinically researched, proven safe and effective weight loss formula here:

http://ProgradeMetabo223x.com

1. Krill Oil:

Supplements with fish oil are an excellent way to get important Essential Fatty Acids (EFA), such as DHA and EPA, which I discussed earlier. Remember, Essential

Fatty Acids such as these may help prevent cancer, heart disease, depression and more. And they can't be produced by the body – we must get EFA from outside sources like food and supplements. This is why we call these fats "essential."

Other Benefits of Taking Krill Oil:

- Improves concentration and memory
- Provides protection for cell membranes
- Aids in healthy nervous system function
- Improves cholesterol
- Supports a strong immune system
- Promotes heart health
- Fights the damaging effects of aging
- **Encourages FAT LOSS!**

Let's discuss that last benefit in greater detail. Not only is krill oil containing EFA important for general health and disease prevention, it's a great way to enhance your fat-burning efforts. That's not to say it's a magic fat-loss pill. Sorry, there's no such thing. However, you can take comfort in knowing that recent studies have shown supplements containing Essential Fatty Acids may have miraculous results.

The enormous health benefits of Essential Fatty Acids have been known for some time, but what's almost startling is the recent research uncovering its weight-loss benefits, as well. In May 2007, a study published in the *American Journal of Clinical Nutrition* reported that a test group incorporating Essential Fatty Acids into their weight-loss plan lost more body fat than all the other test groups in the study combined!

While science hasn't pinpointed exactly why Essential Fatty Acids improve weight loss, I have several theories:

- DHA has been shown to prevent the conversion of pre-fat cells to fat cells, as well as kill pre-fat cells before they become permanent fat cells.

- The EPA and DHA in Krill Oil has the ability to increase both the clearance of chylomicrons (a certain type of fat cell) and fats following a meal. This may have a positive effect on fat usage for energy.

- Essential Fatty Acids can "artificially" decrease heart rate, thus increasing the level of exertion you need to reach a desired exercise intensity. Simply put, you burn more overall calories when exercising.

- Essential Fatty Acids can increase oxidation of fats within fat cells. This means your body burns more fat as energy instead of storing it.

Considering the overwhelming clinical research pointing

to the advantages of EFA supplementation, most weight-loss enthusiasts should be incorporating it into their nutritional plans.

Here is what I recommend: http://Prograde Efa.com

2. Post-Workout Recovery Drink:

Post-workout shakes provide a foundation for accelerated fat loss and recovery after exercise. Research shows that consuming a specific mixture of carbohydrates and proteins enhances recovery of muscle nutrient stores.

How does this affect you? Significant glycogen (i.e., carbohydrate) storage greatly reduces the time it takes your body to recover from exercise. This means you are able to make the most of every workout and burn more calories for fat loss.

In addition to the right kind of carbs, consuming protein immediately after exercise is essential for repairing muscle tissue that has been damaged from exercise (don't worry, this "damage" is a normal part of exercise). Protein also provides the essential amino acids needed to repair muscle tissue so it's ready for your next workout.

Carbs and protein are vital for repairing and preparing your body for the next workout. You should consume a recovery drink within 1 hour of exercise – the sooner, the better. This is the most critical period for replenishing muscle glycogen and amino acid absorption, so you increase lean body mass and burn more calories for weight loss.

If you pass up the proper post-workout nutrition, your exercise performance may suffer the next time you work out. And you may even lose muscle along the way if you don't replenish glycogen and protein quickly.

So what's in a good post-workout supplement? An effective workout recovery drink supplies a blend of high-quality proteins; quick-digesting carbohydrates; free-form amino acids; vitamins; and, finally, essential minerals, including antioxidants to help maximize post-workout recovery. To optimize your training, improve your recovery time, and accelerate fat loss and muscle growth, consume a post-workout drink as part of your training routine.

A Good Post-Workout Drink Contains:

- A formulated 2:1 blend of quick-digesting carbohydrates to protein.
- Protein that's made up of Whey Protein Isolate, which has a concentration higher than 95% protein. Whey Protein Isolate has a very high biological value, meaning it's great for before and after workouts because it's so readily digested, absorbed and used by the body.
- Carbohydrates that consist of dextrose and maltodextrin to facilitate quick absorption and utilization by your muscles.
- The essential B vitamins necessary to provide energy to your cells. This starts the recovery process or fuels cells with energy for upcoming activity.

Recommendation: http://PrograceWorkout.com

3. Multivitamin:

Why do people need to take a multivitamin?

Consistent use of multivitamins and other key supplements can promote good health and help prevent disease, according to a comprehensive new report released by the Council for Responsible Nutrition (CRN).

The report found that ongoing use of multivitamins (preferably those with minerals) and other single-nutrient supplements (like calcium or folic acid) had a positive and quantifiable impact on everything from strengthening elderly patients' immune systems to drastically reducing the risk of neural tube birth defects, such as spina bifida.

This news has relevance for people trying to lose weight, as well. Based on the American Medical Association's recent evaluation of the medical literature, the association recommends Americans consume a one-a-day multivitamin in order to promote general health. Doing so will help you meet your goal to look better and *feel better*.

Health Benefits of Taking a Multivitamin:

- Provides complete daily nutritional supplement foundation
- Provides essential vitamins, minerals, enzymes, amino acids, phytonutrients and whole-food concentrates for optimum health
- Alleviates vitamin deficiencies
- Increases energy levels
- Helps maintain healthy metabolism
- Whole-food base aids assimilation of nutrients

- Supplements any lack of nutrients (e.g., fruits and vegetables) in your diet
- Replaces nutrients depleted by stress

Recommendation:

http://PrograceVGF25.com (for women)

http://PrograceForMen.com (for men)

Chapter 9:

Your New Lifestyle Awaits

Hopefully, you've been measuring your progress throughout this exciting body transformation. I suggest you track your body fat and body circumferences every 3 weeks. Doing so allows you to effectively evaluate whether you need to modify your eating or exercise habits.

Be aware that your progress will change as your transformation continues. At first, you'll see a lot of progress quickly. As you become thinner, that progress will slow down a little. Don't get discouraged and, please, don't obsess over numbers on the scale.

Remember, with proper diet and exercise, you're adding lean muscle at the same time you're losing fat. If you lose 3 lbs of fat, yet gain 3 lbs of muscle, the number on the scale won't budge. But you'll look and feel a whole lot better. And your old dress shirts, T-shirts and jeans will fit a lot looser.

Well, what are you waiting for? If you haven't already,

it's time to start your dramatic body transformation. If you've already used the contents of this book to reach your initial goals – congratulations! You have the rest of your life to enjoy a healthier, slimmer body.

No matter what stage you're at, following the strategies in this book means an exciting new lifestyle is part of your future! Enjoy.

Bonuses

Online Resources:

Weight Loss Made Easy

Quickstart Guide

1. Have you placed your order with ProGrade? Take care of this before anything else in your preparation for Flexible Carb Cycling, as it generally takes a few days for orders to ship and arrive.

We all know the importance of vitamins and minerals and the reality is we do not get in enough of these important nutrients each and every day. Now you know that my motto is food first and to build your nutritional foundation this way. Obviously you can't build a complete foundation through food only due to our lack of variety and depending on where you live the poor nutrient composition of fruits and vegetables.

Another key to your health and potential weight loss success is a high quality fish oil. Right now the recommendation is to eat cold water fish 2-3x a week. This can be challenging for some because they may just not like fish, it gets boring eating fish 3 times a week and again where you live may dictate the level of toxicity that is in the fish.

An easy alternative is taking it in supplement form. This is how nutritional supplements should be used. When used properly you eat well and build a solid foundation and then complete the foundation and fill in the holes and gaps with supplements.

So the 2 most important supplements you should buy right now is http://ProgradeForMen.com, http://ProgradeVGF25.com and http://ProgradeEFA.com. If you want to really accelerate your weight loss results then grab a bottle of Metabo223x.com: http://ProgradeMetabo223x.com

Here is how you can save big. Since I am in charge of R&D for Prograde Nutrition and personally formulate these products, insist on the high quality and production I can also help you save BIG!

The coupon below has a code in it for you to save 20% off the purchase of Prograde products. This is a one time use coupon so I suggest you stock up on the 3 products I mentioned above.

Here is a little secret to save even more. VGF25+, EFA Icon, Metabo 223x and Prograde Protein all have 3 and 6 bottle packages that have big discounts already. You can even get free shipping with the 6 bottle package if you live in the United States or Canada. Well, if you purchase one of those packages you can also save an additional 20% using the coupon code below.

Just enter this coupon code in the shopping cart when checking out.

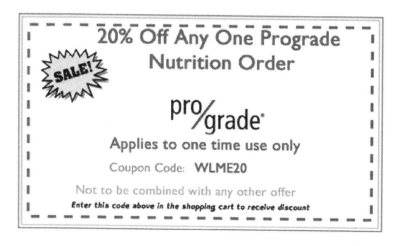

2. Do you have, or have you purchased all the equipment needed to accurately take your measurements? Don't just rely on the scale. It can be very inaccurate when you are strength training and also losing weight.

It is necessary to be consistent when tracking your progress. It is also awesome to know how much fat you have lost and where it was lost from. You can purchase a body circumference measuring tape at most fitness equipment stores or online at http://www.quickmedical.com/fitness/handheld/index.html.

You can find the skinfold calipers at fitness stores or online from a company called Accu-measure:

http://accufitness.com. This company makes a quality pair of skin-fold calipers for a reasonable price.

3. Since you have the necessary tools have you written down your starting stats including your bodyweight, measurements and body fat percentage? Record these in your body fat calculation excel spreadsheet.

   Don't forget to take your "Before" photo for comparison. Probably one of the biggest if not the biggest reason for doing this is because you want to look better. DO NOT SKIP THIS STEP!

4. Have you printed out your meal plans for the first week and purchased the food for that week to start dropping fat? Make sure you go over this and be prepared to add healthy foods to your grocery cart.

5. Did you print out your results journal sheets so you can track each day and the progress you make?

6. Did you check off everything listed above? If so then you are now ready to start the next phase of your life!

Results Journal

This results journal is available for you to print out and make copies. As you can see below it is here for you to be able to record your daily activity and progress. This ensures that you stay on track and focus 100% towards your weight loss goal.

Weight Loss Made Easy Daily Nutrition Assessment

1. Did you plan out your meals in advance?

2. Did you prepare as much as you could ahead of time to avoid excuses and failures?

3. Did you stick to the plan of scheduled meals and quantities of food?

4. Did you avoid off-limits foods?

5. Did you make sure to supplement with Prograde EFA Icon to get in your daily fish (krill) oil requirement?

6. What, specifically, did you fell you did very well on today?

7. What, specifically, about today's eating plan do you feel you can improve upon?

Additional Nutrition Notes:

Weight Loss Made Easy
Daily Exercise Assessment

1. On a scale of 1 - 10, how would you rate your overall activity today?

2. Did you perform either a strength training session or a high intensity cardio interval session today?

3. What can you do to improve your overall activity level to make your weight loss efforts more effective?

Additional Exercise Notes:

Appendix A

Serving Sizes for Food Categories

Starches: Bread, Cereal, Rice, Pastas (80 calories/serving): 1 Carbohydrate Serving =

Food	Serving Size
Angel food cake slice (1 ounce)	1 1/2"
Animal crackers	8
Bagel ounce)	1/2 (1
Baked beans	1/3 cup
Barley, bulgur (cooked)	1/2 cup
Biscuit (2 1/2" across)	1 small
Bran cereal (e.g, Fiber One, All Bran, etc)	1/2 cup
Bread (reduced calorie, lite)	2 slices
Bread (whole wheat, rye, white, pumpernickel)	1

slice

Item	Amount
Breadsticks (4" long by 1/2" across)	4
Broth-based	1 cup
Cake doughnut (plain)	1 small
Chow mein noodles	1/2 cup
Cookies	2 small
Corn (fresh or frozen)	1/2 cup
Corn muffin (2" across) ounces)	1 (2
Corn on the cob ear	1 small
Cornbread (2" square) (2 oz)	1 piece
Couscous (cooked)	1/3 cup
Cream based (low-fat or made with skim milk)	1 cup
Croissant	1 small
Croutons	3/4 cup
Dinner roll ounce)	1 small (1

English muffin ounce)	1/2 (1
French fries (1/2 of a small order)	16 to 25
Frozen yogurt	1/2 cup
Frozen yogurt (fat free)	1/3 cup
Gelatin (sugar sweetened)	1/2 cup
Gingersnaps	3
Graham crackers (2 1/2 inch squares)	3
Grape nuts, muesli, low-fat granola	1/4 cup
Grits	1/2 cup
Hamburger or hot dog bun ounce)	1/2 (1
Hot cereal, cooked (oatmeal, Cream of Wheat, oat bran)	1/2 cup
Ice cream (fat free and no sugar added)	1/2 cup
Matzo ounce	3/4
Melba toast	4
Mixed vegetables with corn, peas, or pasta	1/2 cup

Muffin (cupcake size) ounce)	1 small (1
Oyster crackers	24
Pancake (4" across)	1
Parsnips	1/2 cup
Pasta, cooked (spaghetti, noodles, macaroni) cup	1/3
Peas (green)	1/2 cup
Pita bread (6" across)	1/2
Plantain	1/2 cup
Popcorn (low-fat microwave or popped with no added fat)	3 cups
Potato (baked or broiled) ounces)	1 small (3
Potato (mashed)	1/2 cup
Pretzel sticks ounce	3/4
Pudding (sugar free)	1/2 cup
Pudding (sugar sweetened)	1/4 cup
Puffed cereal (unfrosted)	11/2

cups

Pumpkin	1 cup
Quick bread: banana, pumpkin, zucchini slice (1 ounce)	3/8 inch
Raisin bread	1 slice
Ready-to-eat cereals (e.g., Cheerios, flake cereal, etc.)	3/4 cup
Rice cakes or popcorn cakes (4" across)	2
Rice minicakes or popcorn minicakes	5
Rice, cooked (white or brown)	1/3 cup
Ry-krisp	4
Saltine crackers (2" squares)	6
Sherbet	1/4 cup
Shredded wheat	1 biscuit
Shredded wheat (spoon size, regular or whole wheat)	1/2 cup
Snack chips: tortilla, potato (fat free or baked)	15 to 20
Sorbet	1/4 cup

Stuffing (bread)	1/3 cup
Sugar frosted cereal	1/2 cup
Sweet potato (fresh, without added sugar) mashed, 1 small	1/2 cup
Taco shells, hard (6" across)	2
Tortilla (6" across)	1
Unfrosted cake	2" square
Vanilla wafers	5
Waffle (4" across)	1
Wheat germ	3 TBS
Winter squash (acorn, butternut, buttercup, Hubbard)	1 cup
Yam (fresh, without added sugar) mashed, 1 small	1/2 cup

FAT (45 calories/serving): 1 Fat Serving =

Avocado 1/8 medium avocado	2 TBS or
Bacon fat	1 tsp
Bacon, cooked	1 strip

Butter	1 tsp
Butter, reduced fat	1 TBS
Butter, whipped	2 tsp
Coconut, shredded	2 TBS
Cream cheese	1 TBS
Cream cheese, reduced fat	1 1/2 TBS
Flax oil	1 tsp
Gravy	2 TBS
Half and half (light cream)	2 TBS
Heavy cream	1 TBS
Margarine	1 tsp
Margarine, reduced fat or light	1 TBS
Mayonnaise	1 tsp
Mayonnaise, reduced fat	1 TBS
Miracle Whip salad dressing	2 tsp
Miracle Whip, reduced fat salad dressing	1 TBS
Nondairy cream substitute, liquid or powder	1/4 cup
Nuts (pecans, almonds, or cashews)	4 to 6

Oil (canola, olive, peanut, or sesame)	1 tsp
Olives, black	8 large
Olives, green	10 large
Peanut butter, smooth or crunchy	1/2 TBS
Peanuts	10 large
Salad dress, regular	1 TBS
Salad dressing, reduced fat	2 TBS
Salt pork	1" cube
Seeds, pumpkin, sunflower	1 TBS
Sesame seeds	1 TBS
Shortening or lard	1 tsp
Sour cream	2 TBS
Sour cream, reduced fat	3 TBS
Tahini or sesame paste	2 tsp
Tartar sauce	1 TBS
Tartar sauce, reduced fat	2 TBS
Walnuts	4 halves

Non-Starchy Vegetable Group (25 calories/serving): 1 Vegetable Serving =

Alfalfa   1/2 cup
cooked or 1 cup raw

Artichoke   1/2 cup
cooked or 1 cup raw

Artichoke hearts   1/2 cup
cooked or 1 cup raw

Asparagus   1/2 cup
cooked or 1 cup raw

Bamboo shoots   1/2 cup
cooked or 1 cup raw

Beans (green, Italian, yellow or wax)   1/2 cup
cooked or 1 cup raw

Bean sprouts   1/2 cup
cooked or 1 cup raw

Beets   1/2 cup
cooked or 1 cup raw

Broccoli   1/2 cup
cooked or 1 cup raw

Brussels sprouts   1/2 cup
cooked or 1 cup raw

Cabbage   1/2 cup
cooked or 1 cup raw

Carrots   1/2 cup
cooked or 1 cup raw

Cauliflower   1/2 cup
cooked or 1 cup raw

Celery   1/2 cup
cooked or 1 cup raw

Chicory   1/2 cup
cooked or 1 cup raw

Chinese cabbage   1/2 cup
cooked or 1 cup raw

Cucumber   1/2 cup
cooked or 1 cup raw

Eggplant   1/2 cup
cooked or 1 cup raw

Green onions or scallions   1/2 cup
cooked or 1 cup raw

Greens (beet, collard, dandelion, kale, mustard,
turnip)   1/2 cup
cooked or 1 cup raw

Jicama (Mexican potato)   1/2 cup
cooked or 1 cup raw

Kohlrabi   1/2 cup
cooked or 1 cup raw

Leeks   1/2 cup
cooked or 1 cup raw

Lettuce (endive, escarole, leafy varieties, romaine,
iceberg)   1/2 cup
cooked or 1 cup raw

Mixed vegetables without corn, peas, or pasta 1/2
cup cooked or 1 cup raw

Mushrooms   1/2 cup
cooked or 1 cup raw

Okra   1/2 cup
cooked or 1 cup raw

Onions   1/2 cup
cooked or 1 cup raw

Peppers (all varieties)   1/2 cup
cooked or 1 cup raw

Radishes   1/2 cup
cooked or 1 cup raw

Rhubarb   1/2 cup
cooked or 1 cup raw

Rutabaga   1/2 cup
cooked or 1 cup raw

Sauerkraut   1/2 cup
cooked or 1 cup raw

Snow peas or pea pods   1/2 cup
cooked or 1 cup raw

Spinach   1/2 cup
cooked or 1 cup raw

Summer squash (yellow or green)   1/2 cup
cooked or 1 cup raw

Swiss chard   1/2 cup
cooked or 1 cup raw

Tomato, raw   1/2 cup
cooked or 1 cup raw

Tomato, cherry   1/2 cup
cooked or 1 cup raw

Tomato juice cooked or 1 cup raw	1/2 cup
Tomato paste cooked or 1 cup raw	1/2 cup
Tomato sauce cooked or 1 cup raw	1/2 cup
Turnips cooked or 1 cup raw	1/2 cup
Vegetable juice (e.g., tomato, V8) juice (4 ounces)	1/2 cup
Water chestnuts cooked or 1 cup raw	1/2 cup
Watercress cooked or 1 cup raw	1/2 cup
Zucchini cooked or 1 cup raw	1/2 cup

FRUIT (60 calories/serving): 1 Fruit Serving =

Apple (4 ounces or 2" across)	1 small
Apple, dried	4 rings

Applesauce, unsweetened	1/2 cup
Apricots medium	4
Apricots, canned or frozen, unsweetened	1/2 cup
Apricots, dried	8 halves
Banana (4 ounces)	1/2 small
Blackberries	3/4 cup
Blueberries	3/4 cup
Cantaloupe (1 cup cubed)	1/3 small
Cherries	12 large
Cherries, canned or frozen, unsweetened	1/2 cup
Dates medium	3
Figs, dried medium	1 1/2
Figs, fresh medium or 1 1/2 large	2
Fruit cocktail, canned or frozen, unsweetened	1/2 cup

Fruit juice (100% juice) (4 ounce)	1/2 cup
Grapefruit	1/2 large
Grapes (3 ounces)	17 small
Grapes, canned or frozen, unsweetened	1/2 cup
Guava medium	1
Honeydew melon medium (1 cup cubed)	1/8
Kiwi	1 large
Kumquats medium	5
Mango	1/2 small
Nectarine	1 small
Orange (2 1/2" across, or 6 1/2 ounces)	1 small
Papaya medium (1 cup)	1/2
Passion fruit medium	3

Peach medium	1
Peaches, canned or frozen, unsweetened	1/2 cup
Pear (4 ounces)	1/2 large
Pears, canned or frozen, unsweetened	1/2 cup
Persimmons medium	2
Pineapple, canned or frozen unsweetened	1/2 cup
Pineapple, fresh or canned in own juice	3/4 cup
Plums (5 ounces)	2 small
Plums, canned or frozen unsweetened	1/2 cup
Pomegranate medium	1/2
Prickly Pear	1 large
Prunes medium	3
Raisins	2 TBS
Raspberries	1 cup

Strawberries	11/4 cup
Tangelo medium	1
Tangerines ounces)	2 small (8
Watermelon, cubed	1 1/4 cup

Protein: Meat, Poultry, Fish, Dry Beans, Eggs, Nuts

Lean protein and meat substitutes (0 to 3 grams of fat and 35-55 calories/serving): 1 Lean Protein Serving =

Beef roasts (rib, chuck, rump)	1 ounce
Beef (sirloin, flank, T-bone, porterhouse steak)	1 ounce
Buffalo	1 ounce
Cheese (less than 3 grams of fat per ounce)	1 ounce
Chicken, without skin	1 ounce
Clams	1 ounce
Cornish hen, without skin	1 ounce
Crab	1 ounce

Dried beans, peas, lentils (cooked)	1/2 cup
Duck, without skin	1 ounce
Egg substitute	1/4 cup
Egg whites	2
Elk	1 ounce
Fish (fresh or frozen)	1 ounce
Goose, without skin	1 ounce
Herring	1 ounce
Hot dog, fat free or low fat	1 small
Imitation shellfish	1 ounce
Lamb (roast, chop, leg)	1 ounce
Lobster	1 ounce
Luncheon meat, fat free or low fat	1 ounce
Ostrich	1 ounce
Oysters	1 ounce
Parmesan cheese	2 TBS
Pheasant, without skin	1 ounce
Pork (tenderloin, center loin chop, ham)	1 ounce

Rabbit	1 ounce
Salmon, canned, drained	1 ounce
Sardines medium	2
Scallops	1 ounce
Shrimp	1 ounce
Tuna, canned in water, drained	1 ounce
Turkey, without skin	1 ounce
Veal (roast, lean chop)	1 ounce
Venison	

1 ounce

Medium-fat proteins and/meat substitutes (75 calories/serving): 1 Medium-Fat Protein Serving =

Beef (meatloaf, corned beef, short ribs)	1 ounce
Beef, ground	1 ounce
Cheese (less than 5 grams of fat per serving)	1 ounce

Chicken with skin	1 ounce
Chicken, ground	1 ounce
Cornish hen, with skin	1 ounce
Duck, without skin	1 ounce
Egg	1
Fish, fried	1 ounce
Goose with skin	1 ounce
Lamb (rib roast)	1 ounce
Pheasant, with skin	1 ounce
Pork, ground	1 ounce
Ricotta cheese	1/4 cup
Sausage (less than 5 grams of fat/serving)	1 ounce
Tempeh	1/4 cup
Tofu (soybean curd) (4 ounces)	1/2 cup
Turkey with skin	1 ounce
Turkey, ground	1 ounce
Veal (cutlet)	1 ounce

Whole egg   1

High-fat protein and meat substitutes (100 calories/serving): 1 High-Fat Protein Serving =

Bacon   3 slices

Bratwurst   1 ounce

Cheese (American, cheddar, Colby, Monterey Jack, Swiss)   1 ounce

Cheese spread   2 TBS

Hot dog (turkey, chicken, beef, pork, or combination)
                                                         1

Kielbasa   1 ounce

Luncheon meat (bologna, salami)   1 ounce

Organ meats (liver, heart)   1 ounce

Peanut butter, smooth or crunchy   1 TBS

Pork spareribs, ground pork   1 ounce

Sausage (breakfast)   1 patty or 2 links

Vegetable Protein (Lean) + 1 Starch (115 calories/serving): 1 Serving =

Black beans	1/2 cup
Kidney beans	1/2 cup
Red beans	1/2 cup
Lentils	1/2 cup
Black-eyed peas	1/2 cup
Soy beans (cooked)	1/3 cup
White beans (cooked)	1/2 cup
Garbanzo beans	1/2 cup
Lima beans	1/3 cup
Navy beans	1/3 cup
Split peas	1/3 cup
Pinto beans	1/3 cup

Dairy and Dairy Products (90 calories/serving): 1 Dairy Serving =

Low Fat (90 calories/serving): 1 Low-Fat Dairy Serving =

Cottage cheese (nonfat)	1/2 cup
Buttermilk (fat free or low fat)	1 cup
Dry milk powder (fat free)	1/3 cup
Evaporated skim milk	1/2 cup
Milk (nonfat and 1%)	1 cup
Mozzarella cheese	2 ounces
Pudding (sugar free, made with skim milk)	1/2 cup
Yogurt (fat free, made with sugar substitute)	2/3 cup (6 ounces)
Yogurt (plain, fat free) (6 ounces)	2/3 cup

Reduced-fat (120 calories/serving): 1 Reduced-Fat Serving =

Milk (2%)	1 cup
Natural Cheese	1.5

ounces

Soy milk (plain)	1 cup
Yogurt (plain, reduced fat)	3/4c

Whole-milk products (150 calories/serving): 1 Whole-Milk Serving =

Cottage cheese	3/4 cup
Buttermilk, full fat	1 cup
Evaporated whole milk	1/2 cup
Milk (whole)	1 cup

Free Foods

Beverages

Butter flavoring (fat free)

Carbonated or flavored water (sugar free)

Club soda

Coffee (regular or decaf)

Diet soft drinks (sugar free)

Drink mixes, sugar free

Flavored extracts

Tonic water (sugar free)

Mineral water

Condiments

Garlic

Herbs

Lemon juice Lime juice Mustard

Nonstick pan spray

Pepper

Pimento

Seasonings

Spices

Tea

Vinegar

Water

Wine in cooking

Worcestershire or soy sauce

Miscellaneous

Bouillon or broth
(fat free)
Flavored gelatin
(sugar free)
Gum (sugar free)
Salsa
Sugar substitutes
(aspartame,
saccharin,
acesulfame-K,
etc)
Unflavored
gelatin (plain)

Appendix B

Appendix B is a chart of food exchanges that is very difficult to lay out in a 6x9 printed book.

So to get Appendix B of Food exchange listings go to https://www.mealplans101.com/online-bonuses/

Appendix C

Recipe #1

This is a great recipe for boosting your immune system and cleaning your digestive system.

1 cup fresh whole cranberries

3 apples, seeds removed

Recipe #2:

This is a great drink as a brain booster. It helps you keep your focus and prevent brain fog.

½ large carrot

1 lemon

1 medium cucumber

1 large stalk broccoli, diced up

Recipe #3:

Enjoy this antioxidant powerhouse to rid your body of those free radicals.

2 Granny smith or Gala apples

1 pear

¼ of a large, ripe mango (peel the skin off)

3 strawberries

Recipe #4:

Here is an excellent immune boosting drink to make especially in the winter time.

1 bunch red grapes

1 sweet apple like a Red Delicious

½ medium pomegranate

Dice up the pomegranate with the peel and all before adding it to the blender.

Recipe #5:

Need to cleanse the toxins from your system? Here is the perfect drink for that

2 sweet apples like a Red Delicious

1 knob of fresh ginger (roughly a 1 inch piece)

1 large orange (juice orange like a Valencia)

Recipe #6:

Loaded with Vitamin C, beta carotene and also digestive enzymes

3 strawberries

1 apple

1 mango (peel the skin off and remove the pit)

½ lemon

Recipe #7:

This juice is excellent for reducing inflammation and pain after a hard workout.

1 cup coconut water

½ cucumber

½ red bell pepper

½ apple (remove seed and core from apple)

6 spears asaparagus

½ beet.

Recipe #8:

Boost your alkaline levels with this juice

1 cup kale

1 cup parsley

1 cup spinach

½ cucumber (unwaxed, if you can't find unwaxed cucumbers then peel the skin)

3 celery stalks

½ lemon

2 collard green leaves

Recipe #9:

Attack your free radicals with this probiotic punch.

1 cup spinach

1 cup purple cabbage

2 stalks celery

4 collard leaves

You can add ½ an apple to this if you want to sweeten it up a little.

Recipe #10:

Improve your digestion and mental focus with this booster.

2 cups watermelon

½ lime

1 cup blackberries

small amount of ginger (grated)

Recipe #11:

Get rid of those toxins with this cleanser

2 medium carrots

1 medium cucumber (unwaxed, if you can't find unwaxed cucumbers then peel the skin)

½ large beet

½ head cauliflower

Recipe #12:

This is an excellent juice for cleansing your system and detoxifying.

½ beet

1-2 large carrots

½ unwaxed cucumber (if you can't find unwaxed then peel the skin)

2 collard greens leaves

½ pear

½ lemon

ABOUT THE AUTHOR

Jayson Hunter is an expert in fixing Dysfunctional Fat Cells and helping people lose weight permanently. If you struggle with losing weight then you have Dysfunctional Fat Cells. Through proper nutrient timing of your fat, carbohydrates and protein you not only fix your Dysfunctional Fat Cells, but you lose weight that you are able to keep off for the rest of your life. And while you might initially think this is just some quick weight-loss diet that is ultimately going to leave you disappointed, it isn't. Far from it actually.

Have you ever asked yourself or told yourself:

- Why can't I lose weight even when I don't eat hardly any calories?
- No matter what diet I try I can't seem to lose any weight
- I have a hard time sticking to diets
- Nothing looks good when I am on a diet
- What should I eat to lose weight?

Or have you ever wished that you had someone that would tell you the correct way to lose weight. Where it would be successful and you wouldn't hate following the program or trying to lose weight.

.... You're in the RIGHT place!

As a Registered Dietitian and nationally known weight loss expert that has been seen on ABC, NBC, Fox, and CBS I am the one who **bridges the gap between what science does and what real world living does**.

As a registered dietitian and personal fitness trainer with over 17 years of experience I've seen just about every gimmick, fad diet and miracle pill you may have tried to lose inches fast. And while these "solutions" have worked for the short-term they've resulted in long-term disaster by wreaking havoc on your metabolism. Not only do you gain the weight back you lost, but you gain a whole lot more.

Something very interesting to note is that many of the hundreds of people that I've helped had originally damaged their metabolism through starvation type diets they were using to lose weight for a special occasion. Some wanted to look great for their class reunion. Others wanted to fit into a bikini during their vacation.

The desire to makeover your body needs to be very strong to see results. And when are you going to have a greater desire than when you want to look great for a special day? Or for that vacation you've been wanting to take forever? There's no better time to discover the secrets to not only losing weight fast, but keeping weight off forever!

This information isn't some fad diet filled with nonsense. Everything I reveal to you is based on hard science and research. As a registered dietitian I know what works and what doesn't. I'm not some run-of-the-mill "guru" who pretends to have all the answers. I'm not some well meaning person on an internet forum who wants to help you out. No, I'm a highly educated professional with real-world experience. I do the research and translate it into laymens terms so you can apply it and lose the weight forever.

Instead of digging through hundreds of books, thousands of academic research papers, and wasting time on strategies that you aren't sure work or not let me be the one that does that for you...

And the best part? I'll cut through the fluff, showing you exactly what works and how you can start applying it to your life.

All because I have a knack for breaking down research, apply real life case studies, and everyday life obstacles into INSANELY PRACTICAL TIPS that you can start benefiting from TODAY.

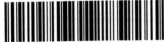

45182743R00094

Made in the USA
San Bernardino, CA
02 February 2017